Telephone Triage and Consultation

Sally-Anne Pygall

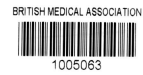

The Royal College of General Practitioners was founded in 1952 with this object:

'To encourage, foster and maintain the highest possible standards in general practice and for that purpose to take or join with others in taking steps consistent with the charitable nature of that object which may assist towards the same.'

Among its responsibilities under its Royal Charter the College is entitled to:

'Diffuse information on all matters affecting general practice and issue such publications as may assist the object of the College.'

British Library Cataloguing-in-Publication Data
A catalogue record for this book is available from the British Library

© Royal College of General Practitioners, 2017
Published by the Royal College of General Practitioners, 2017
30 Euston Square, London NW1 2FB

Designed and typeset by Prepress Projects Ltd, Perth, UK

Printed by Lightning Source UK Ltd

Indexed by Jim Henderson

ISBN 978-0-85084-426-9

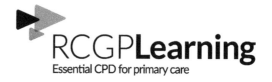

RCGP**Learning**
Essential CPD for primary care

Telephone Triage and Consultation

Are We Really Listening?

Sally-Anne Pygall

Royal College of
General Practitioners

Contents

Contents

Foreword

At a time when our health service is facing ever more unprecedented changes, the increasing challenge for primary care to deliver improved access and safe, effective clinical care to our patients in a climate in which demand now far outweighs capacity means that we must act! We need to adapt our ways of working, ensuring that this is carried out safely and with proper preparation and training. Throughout our medical education and training, we lack formal teaching on telephone triage and consultations. So how do we embark on learning to do this safely and effectively?

Sally-Anne Pygall certainly knows her stuff! This book is a truly essential read for any practice planning to incorporate safe telephone triage into its day-to-day systems. Even if telephone triage is already embedded in your organisation, this excellent resource, written by a clinician with a breadth of first-hand experience in triage systems, will empower you and improve confidence, self-awareness and efficiency. Evidence-based and adopting a sensible step-by-step approach, this book offers the reader an organised, structured account of all of the benefits and inherent risks of telephone triage and provides practical advice on reducing these risks and the importance of communication skills.

In our large, busy, town centre practice we urgently needed to find a practical solution to our increasingly unmanageable patient demand and workload. Sally-Anne's dynamic approach and sound guidance on the use of good telephone triage and consultations has been incredibly effective in helping us to tackle this problem and put us back in the driving seat while improving our patients' access to services and offering them a safe alternative solution to the face-to-face consultation.

This book is an invaluable primary care resource for GPs, trainee GPs, nurses and nurse practitioners. Both those new to general practice and experienced clinicians should read this inspirational and innovative guide, which will undoubtedly help you to acquire the skills needed for safe, efficient telephone triage and consultations.

Dr Samantha Weston
Southport

Preface

The motivation behind this book was to write something that was easily understandable, uncluttered by theory (while acknowledging empirical evidence) and, above all, a real tool that could be used by anyone who was assessing patients over the telephone, whether it be in primary care, secondary care or any other clinical area.

I hope that, in the future, our governing bodies will acknowledge that, as clinicians, we need mandatory formal training in dealing with patients over the phone. It's one of the riskiest areas in which we can work and yet most practitioners haven't had any training – and, by that, I mean good-quality training.

I believe that dealing with patients over the phone could save the health service millions of pounds, but only when it's done well. We could almost abolish the increasing waiting times for appointments to see a general practitioner, reduce outpatient waiting times, improve compliance and therefore reduce admissions – all by using the phone more effectively and safely. Ministers take note.

The advent of 'online consultations' is worrying, in my opinion – and I hope you will agree once you have read this book and understand the importance of really listening. If you can't even hear the patient or carer, there is so much that you could miss.

I fervently hope that this book will help you understand how you can help patients without always having to see them, and when the risk of not seeing someone is unacceptable, or when more urgency is required than you may have previously realised. Telephone work can be totally rewarding and liberating and, above all, can help provide a better health service for our patients.

About the author

Sally-Anne Pygall runs the only company currently in the UK specialising in training and consultancy services in telephone triage and consultations for clinicians and telephone skills for non-clinicians. As a senior nurse with decades of experience in telephone health care, Sally-Anne is a fervent advocate of telephone triage, having worked in the NHS, the private sector and social enterprise organisations. She has gained a wealth of experience and knowledge, unrivalled in telephone health care. She delivers training on telephone skills on behalf of the RCGP, clinical commissioning groups, universities, vocational training schemes and out-of-hours providers and also provides services as an expert witness, but her main area of training is within general practice.

Sally-Anne has an MSc in Evidence Based Practice from York University and has run her own company since 2009.

Telephone health care carries considerable risks for everyone involved, and Sally-Anne understands better than most how ill prepared many clinicians are to undertake this specialist skill. Her passion for telephone triage and consultations and her aspiration to educate clinicians to carry out safe and effective triage is her greatest motivation. Sally-Anne is married with two sons and lives in the north-east of England.

Acknowledgements

I would like to thank the RCGP for giving me the opportunity to write this book, which has been years in the making – if only I'd realised it! It's been a painful, but extremely rewarding, process, which has made me question my own knowledge on a subject that I knew I was passionate about before – and am even more so now.

This book, however, could not have been written without the help of several people: Gillian Nineham, to whom I am extremely grateful for talking sense to me and approaching me in the first place about writing the book. I would never have had the courage otherwise to get it done if you hadn't given me the confidence and assistance. Thank you.

To Dr Andy Parsons and Dr Himanshu Gupta: your encouragement, honesty and help in reviewing my work has been invaluable. Whenever I needed a kick up the proverbial backside, a swift talking to, a helping hand or just a sounding board, you were there. Most of all, your words of reassurance meant more than you could ever know. Thank you both.

To Kathryn Martin: thank you for your help and support.

To those clinicians who have challenged me in training, who have questioned my capability and made me doubt myself, I thank you too. It's this kind of testing that has pushed me to find out more and have confidence. I hope that, by reading this book, you will see and hear what I may not have had the opportunity to say when we met.

Finally, I need to thank my husband, Christian, and our sons. There have been times when I wasn't with you because I needed to write and times when I know I must have bored you immeasurably rattling on about this book. I love you and thank you all very much.

Introduction

It has become increasingly obvious that the NHS (National Health Service) cannot continue to sustain a primary care service in which a consumerist approach to health care is becoming progressively evident. In the last few years, we have seen some dramatic changes in how we deliver health care, changes that some clinicians and patients have embraced and others have maligned. One of the most significant transformations is the increasing use of the telephone in patient care. Telephone contact is the first step on the patient care pathway for accessing out-of-hours (OOH) services, for example, while internationally telephone triage is now commonly the first point of contact for health services in many countries including the USA, Denmark, Canada, Australia and Sweden.

In the UK, many surgeries are also moving to a more telephone-led delivery model as a means of improving access and managing demand. However, many GPs (general practitioners) and nurses carrying out health care by telephone have not been formally trained in making assessments over the phone. Reassuringly, several training institutions are now recognising the need to prepare healthcare professionals for what is a very challenging clinical skill.

This book is suitable for anyone dealing with patients over the phone, but it's principally aimed at GPs and nurses working in primary care, in both general practice and OOH settings. It seeks to provide the reader with a practical and real-world approach to telephone triage and consultations. A telephone assessment is not just about using an evidence-based systematic approach to triage and consultation – it's also about how you communicate with your caller, knowing when – and when not – to rely on the information you have gathered in the absence of visual or physical examination. Ultimately it's about making sure that patients are safe – whether or not you are seeing them.

Patients can be harmed as a result of poor telephone triage, and many clinicians are nervous about undertaking it, as they realise how difficult and demanding it can be and prefer the 'safety' of seeing patients. However, this book will give readers a real understanding of how to carry out telephone assessments to minimise the risks to the patient, as well as themselves, and, more importantly, how to recognise when patients should be seen, rather than attempting to help them over the phone.

One of the biggest condemnations of telephone triage is that it can lead to a 'misdiagnosis', which in turn can lead to an inappropriate or adverse outcome for the patient. Uniquely, the aim of this book is to show that it is more relevant to think of this as a 'mistriage' rather than a misdiagnosis. This book will strive to teach the clinician the importance of getting the triage or consultation right, rather than concentrating on determining the diagnosis.

Throughout this book, the term 'caller' will refer to the person who requests a call back, or contacts a clinician for advice via the telephone. This can be the patient or someone ringing on behalf of the patient. Although some calls can be arranged by the clinician to follow up on previous contact, in this book the term 'caller' will always refer to the patient or carer, and not the clinician.

The style of writing used within the book is distinctively conversational, rather than taking a more formal prose approach, and, although there will be references to research, the book should be seen as a very practical guidebook, with a style of writing that reflects this realistic approach. This is intended to be your 'how to' manual – one that is based on empirical evidence but, more importantly, founded in real-life experience and knowledge of telephone triage and consultations. I hope that readers will return to it time and time again for sensible advice on how to take a call.

Chapter 1

Telephone triage and consultations: their purpose, benefits and risks

1.1 Telephone triage versus telephone consultations – is there a difference?

OK, let's deal with this question straight away. Have you picked up this book because you want to know about telephone triages or about telephone consultations? Do you think there is a difference? Do you think you are doing one but not the other, or that you move from one to the other as required, or have you set up your systems to address both? In this section I will attempt to convince you that there really is no difference between how we act when taking a 'triage' call compared with conducting a 'consultation', but, if you are not convinced, I would ask you to accept this concept in principle, as the terms *triage* and *consultation* will be used interchangeably throughout this book.

First, I think we need to clarify that some of the phone calls that you will be dealing with should be considered neither a consultation nor a triage, as no form of assessment takes place.

For instance, telephone calls that are not a consultation or a triage might include:

- requests for repeat sick notes
- providing routine or normal test results
- repeat prescription requests
- any call in which there are no clinical questions asked
- requests for letters or forms for insurance purposes or legal matters.

I hope you would agree that these types of calls are neither a triage nor a consultation: they take in some cases less than a minute and there is no clinical 'discussion' or advisory element.

When an assessment occurs and where the outcome is not predetermined – that is what I believe should be considered a triage or a consultation, and those are the calls that this book will address. Generally, these calls are initiated by the caller or patient, but not exclusively, as they may also include 'reviews' that involve an element of assessment of current symptoms. If you really think about it, what happens during both types of calls, however, is exactly the same – you ask some questions to find out how the patient is, what seems to be wrong and then decide whether he or she should be seen or not and, if so, how quickly. Your actions as a clinician are the same – *so isn't a telephone triage therefore the same as a telephone consultation and vice versa?* Let's examine the potential variances further to see how a triage may differ from a consultation.

How is a telephone consultation defined?

Most of us will understand what is meant by the term 'telephone consultation', i.e. it refers to an in-depth clinical assessment of a patient via the phone, and it also applies when patients or carers communicate with someone in a healthcare profession about a health problem or enquiry. They are often pre-booked by either the patient or the clinician, or perhaps used for a follow-up review rather than a face-to-face consultation. A telephone consultation may be given an actual appointment time and allocated several minutes – perhaps even the same length of time as a face-to-face consultation – and is often thought to negate the need to see the patient. Typically, telephone consultations are thought to take more time than telephone triages.

How is telephone triage defined?

Telephone triage has been defined as 'prioritising client's health problems according to their urgency, educating and advising clients and making safe, effective and appropriate decisions'.[1] It has also been defined as 'sorting patients into order of priority for treatment'[2] or 'the action of sorting according to quality'.[3] We use triage within many healthcare sectors to identify what is urgent, what can wait and what needs to happen next, so face-to-face triage is often the forerunner of other care. In other words, patients are not commonly 'discharged' at this point, although of course some may be, but the triage usually leads to an additional assessment or care episode. Telephone triage is different from other forms of triage, however, 'as there is no physical patient presence and therefore no examination is possible'.[4] It is expected to be a rapid and brief determination of what care a patient requires, or a way of managing some of the non-acute work mentioned earlier. 'Telephone triage' is a term frequently used when a phone call is arranged as a result of running out of appointments, and for managing the 'overflow', as a quick (and, let's face it, sometimes dirty) signposting and prioritisation, or as a system for managing the demand for same-day appointments.

Does a telephone triage usually result in an additional care episode, as would be the case for a patient who may have been triaged in an emergency department, or can a telephone triage be the end of a care episode? Yes, it most certainly can, and indeed it should be in at least 50% of cases (more on those figures later). Telephone triage *is* different from face-to-face triage though: you wouldn't say to a patient, 'Sorry but this initial phone call is just to ask you what's been happening and, now that I know what it sounds like, you will require a second phone call, as I have determined from the triage that you now need a consultation', would you? The models that apply to face-to-face triage are designed to be used when you can see and touch the patient and are not therefore reliably transferable to telephone triage.

What might the differences between telephone triage and consultations look like in reality, if you still think they are different? You may have a call about a potential emergency, for example, when a patient has reported chest pain. After talking on the phone, however, you find out that the pain is localised, the patient is totally well otherwise, there are no other red flags and it was brought about by an activity, which leads to a diagnosis of musculo-skeletal pain. You do not need to send an ambulance and you may not even need to see the patient, as it's certainly not an emergency and you are confident in your diagnosis. The 'triage' has resulted in self-care management. It has taken you several minutes to determine what was actually happening and how unwell (or not) your patient is and to give the appropriate advice for managing self-care. This call now appears to be more like what you would expect from a 'consultation', doesn't it, but you wouldn't say to the patient, 'Sorry. I need to arrange a consultation now'.

Alternatively, a telephone consultation could typically be arranged when a female patient reports symptoms of a urinary tract infection, but it could quickly develop into a critical situation after you find out that she has atypical abdominal pain. She may even be dehydrated and require urgent attention. The 'consultation' has turned into what you might think of as a 'triage', i.e. very much shorter and with an urgent outcome. The beginning of nearly every consultation has to include an initial triage to make sure that the patient doesn't need a rapid response and a triage may result in a full-length interaction resulting in self-care management. Therefore, *aren't they potentially all triages or all consultations?* You don't actively switch from one type of clinical assessment style to another do you?

The number of questions you ask, however, and the amount of time you devote to a call may be predetermined as a result of your attempt to deal with something quickly (a triage) or if a patient has requested a phone call (a consultation). Your outcome can often be dependent on how quickly *you* want to deal with a call, or by whether you think the patient is expecting a longer interaction. More interestingly, I have found that the *outcome is often decided by*:

- the access you have available, i.e. number of appointments or home visits already booked
- the time of day
- who will be seeing the patient following the telephone call (some clinicians are more hesitant about having patients seen if they are adding to someone else's workload, but less so if it is their own workload they are adding to)
- whether you have already run out of appointments (you might be less likely to see someone if there are fewer appointments available)
- whether you are taking calls at the end of the day (you might be less likely to want to see your patient if you want to go home on time)
- whether you want to go home without worrying about someone you didn't see (you are more likely to see that person)
- your concurrent level of mental acuity
- whether you are tired and/or stressed.

So, what really happens is that you have all of these factors influencing how you decide to manage the call. In my experience, *many patients are seen not because they have to be seen from a clinical perspective but simply because they can be seen, and many outcomes are determined by workload and the availability of appointments.*

So, is there a difference between a triage and a consultation? In my opinion there isn't – or, at least, there shouldn't be – as your role is to ask enough questions to find out what is best for the patient. Your outcomes should not be influenced by what access is available but by what the patient needs clinically. This may take only a few seconds or several minutes, no matter whether you are doing a 'triage' or a 'consultation'. More importantly, if you want your phone interactions to be successful, you may need to rethink your approach to your decision making and look at the clinical need first, then patient choice, alongside access options. Understanding and adhering to this simple strategy could change how you do telephone work.

I hope that I have convinced you that there is no difference between a telephone triage and a telephone consultation when it comes to the practicalities of taking a call. In short, it refers to the process of the clinical assessment carried out over the phone and, as mentioned earlier, I will use the terms interchangeably in the rest of this book.

How do we make decisions in telephone triage?

There are some interesting similarities between the processes of telephone triage and air traffic control,[5] in which the psychological processes of identifying and solving diagnostic problems within a time-constrained environment drives complex decision making. These decisions have to be made within seconds at times in both cases, as lives can be at stake. Perhaps the key difference, however, is in the matter of patient or 'passenger' involvement. The air traffic controller does not ask whether the passenger agrees with his or her instructions but rather makes all decisions independently of the concerns of the passenger and perhaps even the pilot. In telephone triage, the concerns, ideas and expectations of the patient and carer play a major role in the outcome of and advice given during the consultation.

The definition of telephone triage I like the most, however, is its description as 'decision making under conditions of uncertainty and urgency'.[6] This definition is very apt, as the uncertainly of not being able to see patients has a dramatic impact on your confidence; you cannot make those initial assessments about their general condition as you would when you first see them in the surgery or your place of work. It has been hypothesised that doctors can diagnose patients within 30 seconds[7] – this is partly because they can see and smell them and determine whether the first words spoken by a patient support their initial visual assessment. With experience, a doctor or nurse can often tell you what is wrong with someone just by looking at him or her, especially where there is an existing relationship. Without the initial visual and olfactory information, you may understandably feel very unsure. However, with continued experience of telephone triage, you will learn to replace those visual clues with auditory ones and you may even be a better diagnostician because of it. It is easy to rely too much on what you see, rather than what the patient or carer is telling you – they say so much without putting it into words, but *are you really listening?*

Our uncertainty as clinicians when we cannot confirm information visually is reasonable, but equally important, however, is the fact that the patient cannot see the triager. As clinicians, there is a tendency to think more of how our ability to work is affected by the loss of the visual information, and we may forget the patients' experience and what they are missing. It is difficult for some patients to accept that we can care for them when we haven't seen them. Much of our own uncertainty of telephone triage leads to a lack of confidence and sometimes an overwhelming need to see the patient, when it really isn't necessary.

As has also been suggested, there is often a degree of urgency to telephone triage,[6] not only from a clinical perspective where an emergency response may be required but also because telephone triage is commonly allocated less time than a face-to-face consultation. This is ironic when you consider that you cannot make those initial visual assessments (and diagnostic assumptions) that occur within the first minute or so of a face-to-face consultation. It could be argued that you actually require more time for telephone triage, as you may also lack any patient history. For example, in out-of-hours work, i.e. when the surgery is closed, the patient's notes are often unavailable, and the clinician must ascertain the patient's relevant past medical history, medications, etc., as well as current or acute history during the call, thereby adding to the consultation time. When you are working within a total triage system (see Chapter 10), i.e. one in which almost *all* patients will be taken through a telephone call before an appointment for a face-to-face consultation is made, the number of calls a clinician may deal with in a single session can be enormous. This can place terrific pressure on the triager to deal with the calls as quickly as possible. The shortest call I have personally ever heard to date was 21 seconds long, and here it is (this is the call in full):

> *Doctor: Hello, it's the doctor here. What's the problem?*
> *Patient: Oh, I have stomach pains.*
> *Doctor: Mmm, hmm.*
> *Patient: Yes, since 1 o'clock in the afternoon.*
> *Doctor: OK, come down to the surgery (names urgent care centre)*
> *Patient: Where?*
> *Doctor: (names urgent care centre again)*
> *Patient: Oh, OK.*
> *Doctor: Mmm. (puts, or rather slams, phone down)*

I hope you will see how dangerous this type of call is. It would take me several paragraphs to point out what was wrong, but if you are tempted to think that this is an 'efficient' way of managing something that typically would require a face-to-face consultation, consider that we have no idea how ill the patient is and, if it turned out that she didn't attend at all, it would probably be classed as a 'Did Not Attend' when it could be that she collapsed and died (or, of course, simply decided not to bother).

The urgency, however, may also come from your callers in some cases, as they may want you to deal with them as quickly as possible, or they don't want to go through a lot of questions, therefore making you 'rush' the interaction.

Many studies show that healthcare professionals value the telephone as a convenient method of managing patient demand and workload. More recent studies, however, have also raised questions over its use for acute illnesses and whether telephone consultations include sufficient information to exclude serious illness.[8,9] This may be because less time is allocated to the interaction than to a face-to-face consultation and that is why there could be insufficient information available. It's not uncommon to see only 3 minutes on average allocated to telephone triages. How safe is that when you cannot confirm things visually or physically? What impact does it have on the triagers when they are under that kind of time pressure? We will discuss this later in this chapter.

1.2 What are the benefits of telephone care?

Telephone triage and consultations (remember, we will use these terms interchangeably to refer to a clinical assessment of a patient's needs over the phone) have many benefits for the patient, the carer, the healthcare provider and healthcare organisations, *but* only when they are done well. It would be foolish to assume that you will inherit all the benefits simply by offering telephone triage. If it is not performed correctly, it will not yield the benefits, will increase the risks and could significantly increase workload.

If we start with the patient and/or the carer, telephone consultations offer the following benefits.

- *Immediate access in some cases.* Being able to talk to a clinician (sometimes within minutes) is very attractive to some patients or their carers. In today's society, which is very consumer driven, with the expectation of instant gratification, patients and carers have now begun to expect the same level of immediate service from healthcare providers. Even within the NHS, as opposed to private healthcare societies, patients are encouraged by politicians to expect care within very short time frames. This has been one of the most dramatic changes in primary health care over the last decade: the time patients expect to wait before seeing their GP. Patients demand access almost immediately (inappropriately, in many cases) and, by providing telephone access, many organisations are able to meet a lot of this demand.

- *Easier, more convenient access.* Many patients find it more convenient to speak to their care provider over the phone, as they can speak to someone wherever they are, e.g. at work, at home, while travelling or shopping, etc. Alternatively, they don't have to take time off work to see someone or try to book an appointment on their only day off (often a major cause of dissatisfaction with limited appointments available). Many private healthcare organisations are now offering telephone support to people travelling abroad, or they provide access to prescription medication that can be delivered to the patient's door following a telephone conversation, rather than the patient (or client) having to travel to a clinic for assessment and treatment.

- *Opportunities for patient education and empowerment.* One of the greatest benefits of telephone care is the opportunity to educate patients so that they are empowered to manage their own health care, or have a better understanding of when they really need to see their GP, so that they are not making appointments unnecessarily or inappropriately. Studies comparing GP triage with nurse triage in primary care[10] have suggested that nurses may make longer phone calls because they spend more time offering patients education. By educating the patient or caller they can have more confidence in managing the problem themselves. Furthermore, by knowing the disease trajectory, the caller may not jump in to make a second contact when things don't immediately improve. Studies have also suggested that telephone reviews aid compliance in long-term conditions such as asthma.[11]

- *May avoid the need for a face-to-face consultation.* Studies have suggested that up to 50% of patients in primary care can be managed safely over the phone.[12,13] When telephone triages are done safely and efficiently, avoiding a face-to-face consultation can improve access overall, as more patients can be dealt with. Surgeries in which total triage is the service delivery model (see Chapter 10) are dealing with two or three times as many patients over the phone as they previously would have in face-to-face consultations, but are only seeing perhaps 25–40% of those patients face to face following the phone call. The second interaction in the surgery should, by default, be shorter (when the triager is also the face-to-face clinician), but again all of this depends on the quality of the triage. Many practices will implement a telephone system of assessment to avoid seeing as many patients, but, if the triage is not effective, there will be no reduction in face-to-face consultations, or the triage can become unsafe.

- *Cost savings.* By not having to travel to the surgery, patients or carers can save on travel costs and, if they can have their prescriptions delivered, this is an even more attractive way of accessing health care. Alternatively, if patients pay for their health care, it could be a much less costly way of accessing health advice. However, if the GP receives fees only for 'seeing patients' (as can be the case in Australia, for instance), there is no incentive for the GP to offer telephone consultations or to provide advice or treatment without seeing the patient, and so there is little benefit.
- *Reduced carbon footprint.* With today's concerns about climate change, we need to consider the environment and how it can be affected by having people travel by car or bus unnecessarily. It is relevant to consider that, by avoiding a trip to the surgery, patients and carers are reducing their carbon footprint and helping protect the environment.

For the healthcare provider (GP, nurse, emergency care practitioner, etc.), the benefits include the following.

- *Cost-effective services.* Telephone triages can reduce the number of face-to-face GP appointments required (by 50% or more). According to the *Unit Costs for Health and Social Care 2015*,[14] a face-to-face consultation with a GP takes an average of 11.7 minutes, whereas a telephone consultation takes an average of 7.1 minutes, so there is a saving of 4.6 minutes per patient. This should mean that GPs could deal with more patients, as well as give time to other activities that may be more beneficial to other patients, or to GPs themselves. Alternatively, GPs may be able to reduce the costs of locum cover, where the demand for appointments has escalated; thousands of pounds spent on locum cover can be significantly reduced, and perhaps even entirely eliminated, by dealing with more patients over the phone. I know of one surgery that saved almost £150,000 in locum costs after implementing the total triage system. By triaging requests for home visits (the costliest of services, as each visit requires on average 30 minutes), you can significantly reduce the number of visits made. Even a saving of one visit a week can add up to an extra 2 or 3 working days a year! It must be said, nonetheless, that recent studies have suggested that there is little cost saving, as the workload is simply redistributed rather than reduced. However, these studies do not indicate the quality of the actual triage or how it was judged as being 'appropriate' or not as far as outcomes are concerned. There is no mention of the use of a quality assurance tool (see Chapter 8) to assess the quality of the calls or whether the judgement was based on listening to the call, reviewing the documentation or both. This is vitally important when making decisions about models of care. As I have said previously – simply doing telephone triage is not the benefit – the benefit comes from good triage. If nurse triage can replace GP triage (while maintaining the quality), that can result in simple cost savings.

- *More appropriate use of resources.* Many practices now employ nurses to carry out telephone triage for minor illnesses and acute same-day demand, for instance. This can significantly increase GPs' availability and allow them to deal with the more complex conditions. Following on from the triage, the patient may be seen by a more appropriate practitioner, e.g. a nurse rather than a GP, thereby making a second saving. It may become clear that the best person to deal with the patient is someone outside the usual practice team, e.g. a pharmacist, physiotherapist, social worker, mental health care support team member, A&E (accident and emergency department) and many more. Good triage will also ensure that patients are seen when they really need to be seen and that GPs and nurses are dealing with those patients who require medical assistance within the practice rather than the worried well.

- *Managing surgery workload by prioritising patients.* Many patients who need to be seen don't need to be seen urgently and can be offered a routine appointment rather than being squeezed in at the end of a session. Alternatively, you may decide that a patient should be seen urgently and by having fewer face-to-face consultations, this can be arranged more easily. Finally, some patients should be seen by the emergency services by calling 999 or attending A&E rather than visiting the surgery at all.

- *Reducing the cycle of inappropriate access to scheduled and unscheduled care.* By triaging patients on the phone prior to their attending their GP or making an unscheduled visit, a substantial amount of inappropriate access could be reduced, or even avoided altogether. I was once told of a surgery that implemented a total triage system that involved patients being assessed by any of the GPs on duty that day. This approach led to many of the patients of one particular GP being triaged by his colleagues.

The GP in question was usually fully booked weeks in advance before the triage system was introduced, but when his patients were then being dealt with by other GPs, they realised that this particular GP was practising very little medicine and dealing with less complex, and often less demanding, patients. He was actively encouraging patients to see him, and him alone, and was having nice little chats with them, taking blood pressures, and so on. He was responsible for a lot of the unnecessary access. Furthermore, a cardiologist once told me that, as clinicians, we can very often turn 'people' into 'patients' and, by seeing patients unnecessarily, we encourage a cycle of accessing care.

- *Improving compliance with treatment for long-term conditions through telephone reviews.* Studies have suggested that telephone reviews aid compliance in long-term conditions such as asthma.[11] The telephone is a convenient way of reviewing patients without them having to take time off work. Many younger patients have a mobile phone with them at all times, so, by having more timely reviews that don't involve a trip to the surgery, patients can be advised to implement treatment much earlier and therefore avoid a crisis or the need for hospital treatment. Post-surgical reviews can be carried out over the phone, which reduces the number of outpatient appointments required and is more convenient for patients. Wherever you work, really think about the benefits you might be able to achieve through telephone assessments or reviews and then weigh up those benefits against the risks before you decide whether this method of patient care is right for you. Remember, though, that we are looking at the benefits of *good* triage and not just any telephone triage, as poor triage can negate any benefits and increase risks. So, what about the risks?

1.3 What are the risks of telephone triage?

Decision making in telephone triage is associated with high levels of risk because of the complex decision-making processes involved and the context of the setting, i.e. primarily busy services with staff and resource constraints. It could be compared in many ways to other environments, as discussed earlier, such as air traffic control and emergency service dispatching, where rapid and precise decisions are necessary. It is also affected by the patient or caller's level of comprehension in providing the information necessary for the triager to gain an accurate clinical picture of the problem.

Knowing where the risks may lie and how those risks can be managed (or not, as the case may be) will determine whether telephone triage is right for you and the patient. Although I am a huge advocate of telephone care, there are times when it is not the best way of dealing with patients, as the risks outweigh the benefits.

Some of the risks you will need to be aware of are listed below.

- *Assumptions!* This is probably the riskiest thing to do – make an assumption during a call. Many telephone triages fail, as the triager or the caller has assumed that they understood something. They didn't check out their understanding with the other person, or either person assumes that they are being understood when they are not. *Never assume anything when you cannot confirm it visually or physically.* Something as simple as understanding where a point of pain is can be completely incorrect if you assume that the person is describing it accurately, or understands where the parts of the body are. For example, the location of the kidneys is notorious for being described inaccurately! Another example is when someone may think that the pain is in their back, when it is actually in the upper chest, or 'stomach pain' is in fact chest pain. I have heard many calls that have ended in very poor outcomes that arose because of an assumption, which then led to a mistriage and therefore a misdiagnosis and incorrect decision making.
- *The lack of visual clues can lead to uncertainty and inappropriate outcomes.* So let's state the obvious – because you can't see the patient it is easier to get it wrong. Many clinicians are reluctant to carry out telephone triage, as they feel safer when they can see the patient, but, in today's healthcare system, this approach may be unsustainable, and so clinicians are doing telephone triage even when they are very nervous about it. They struggle to get past not being able to see, touch or smell their patient and many go on to arrange a face-to-face consultation when it isn't necessary. More worryingly, some clinicians do not appreciate the difficulties of telephone triage and approach it with a blasé attitude, deciding that someone doesn't need to be seen when they really should be – and quickly. It is also possible to refer patients to a higher level of care such as A&E when they could have been managed in primary care. In all of these cases, the lack of visual confirmation leads to a degree of uncertainty that can easily result in an inappropriate outcome; one of the biggest risks of all is delaying, or even denying, a face-to-face consultation with a patient.
- *You are reliant on the caller for an accurate recall of history.* The level of comprehension of the caller plays a significant part in the interaction, and poor comprehension levels could result in mistriage. In some cases, the

caller may also fail to present information that could affect the outcome. For example, when you ask the simple question, 'Do you have any medical history that I need to know about?', callers will often answer negatively, and yet, when questioned about medications, they will reel off a list as long as your arm! Other patients have trouble remembering the names of medications or conditions and it becomes a piece of detective work to put all the pieces together, before deciding how relevant the information is. If the triager suspects that the caller is not reliable in terms of giving an accurate recall of the history, it will probably be safer to arrange a face-to-face consultation, but still take account of the urgency. In some cases, failure to present accurate information has nothing to do with comprehension levels – it's just that the question was poorly phrased in the first place and the caller is struggling to make sense of it. A caller may also be unable to adequately express or describe the problem, or perhaps it is a third party that did not witness the incident, e.g. a mother who picks up her young child from somewhere and is told that 'he banged his head', so she can't give you an accurate or detailed explanation of how the injury occurred, as she wasn't there. One of the biggest problems will be due to differences in language. This really is about stating the obvious – if you don't speak the same language, how reliable is either the information given by the caller or the understanding of the information by the triager? We will pick this up again in Chapter 2.

- *Third-party calls.* That is someone calling on someone else's behalf, such as a parent calling on behalf of a child or an adult calling on behalf of an elderly relative. Although it can be necessary to triage through a third party, when you don't speak directly with patients, you lose a great deal of your initial assessment, such as how they sound (i.e. generally unwell or well) or what their breathing is like, for example. There is a higher risk of gaining inaccurate information from a third party, which can lead to a wrong outcome (too high or too low a level of care). Third-party callers may overplay or underplay symptoms – typically, parents can overplay their child's illness, whereas elderly patients often underplay how ill they are to a relative or carer. The third party can make assumptions or miss something entirely, and cases of 'Chinese whispers' are not uncommon, but the bigger risk is when the third party is not with the patient at the time of the call (see Chapter 6) and so is unable to check on the patient and/or the symptoms contemporaneously, thereby doubling the risk. Triaging through a third party when it isn't necessary can lead to mistriage and misdiagnosis.

- *Inappropriate face-to-face appointments may be given.* This increases dependence, delays someone else's care and increases workload. It might be difficult to accept how seeing patients who don't really need to be seen is a risk, but, for patients themselves, there is a risk of increasing dependency. They can begin to feel that you need to see them at all times to 'care' for them. This isn't true in a lot of cases – not seeing patients doesn't mean that you aren't caring for them or that a telephone consultation is a second-class service. If patients have traditionally been seen, however, it can be difficult to persuade them that they don't need this later. If one clinician carries out a triage and opts for a face-to-face consultation when it wasn't necessary, and then the same patient speaks to someone else, who suggests that the patient self-manages, or doesn't need to be seen that day, the patient can easily think, 'But I was seen straight away last time I called!'. Protracted negotiation can ensue about what needs to happen and why. The second triager is then facing an uphill battle from the start, because of the previous outcome and the patient's expectations. When patients who don't need to be seen take up an appointment, it can mean that other patients, who really do need to be seen, end up waiting much longer than they needed to; the risk isn't to the patient being triaged but to other patients. If patients can't get to see the GP or nurse when they need to be seen because there are no appointments available, they may attend other resources, such as A&E, when it is neither an accident nor an emergency, thereby adding to costs for the GP and clinical commissioning group. Finally, some patients make frequent but unnecessary contacts, and if these contacts then result in inappropriate appointments, there is a risk that the clinician is overworked and risks burnout. Burnout due to increased work load is amplified when clinicians are nervous about not seeing patients.
- *Poor communication or poor interaction.* 'Poor communication' on the phone can mean many things, and it can be subjective, which is why I have dedicated a whole chapter of this book to communication skills. However, some poor communication and therefore poor interaction is due to a lack of engagement. This results in inaccurate information gathering, complaints and the potential to mistriage. Communicating effectively is a major feature in risk management. A considerable number of complaints are not as a result of a clinical concern, but simply because the callers did not like the way they were spoken to or the 'attitude' of the triager.

- *Patients may perceive telephone triage as reducing access to care.* If patients aren't sure about telephone triage and don't understand what you can do for them over the phone, some may see a triage system as reducing their access to GPs, especially where each face-to-face consultation with a GP or nurse must first begin with a telephone call (the total triage model). They can view it as an unnecessary hoop that they must jump through to get what they perceive they need – to be seen. If patients are against telephone triage, they will be less inclined to accept both the service and the advice or outcome. Preconceived ideas and expectations will be a difficult barrier to overcome and the consequences can be an inappropriate conclusion, but they are not impossible to avoid.

- *Poor documentation and record keeping.* Here, I am referring to the electronic or paper record, *not* voice recording, and I have seen enormous variations among individuals and teams. Sometimes, it can be very sparse documentation (especially when the triager is arranging to see the patient), as the clinician intends to do a full-length documentation following the face-to-face consultation. Other times (more so when the outcome is self-care management), the documentation can go on and on, with every part of the conversation written in protracted detail. In Chapter 7 we will cover this risk in more detail, but, suffice to say, if your documentation is lacking and something goes wrong, you will open yourself up to legal liability. A second risk factor is that, when it comes to recall, there is research that suggests that the brain is better at remembering visual information rather than audio or written information.[15] If you are ever asked to recall and justify an outcome, your record keeping will be crucial, but, if that record keeping is poor or inadequate, your ability to cite the interaction may be made much harder, owing to the absence of visual cues as a prompt.

- *Some patients dislike it.* Some patients will always prefer a face-to-face consultation rather than a phone conversation, not because they don't trust this method of caring for them but just because they like to see the person they are talking to. There are still lots of people who would always prefer a face-to-face conversation to a telephone conversation, so if their practice utilises a total triage system, they won't like it and this can lead to complaints and dissatisfaction.

- *Time constraints.* Perhaps I should have placed this risk at the very top, as it is, in my opinion, one of the greatest problems with telephone triage in busy services – the issue of not having enough time. Now, this time pressure can be generated internally (from the clinician and their workload) or externally (by the caller). In the case of the former, many clinicians find themselves taking calls in between seeing patients and so want to get the call done as quickly as possible, or at the end of surgery when they have a mountain of other work to do, such as administration work and/or home visits. Where total triage is being delivered, surgeries may have allocated only 3 minutes per call. Where this happens, the natural reaction for the clinicians, whether consciously or not, is to try to complete the call as quickly as they can. When you are under time pressure, you risk any, or all, of the following things happening: untimely conclusion; lack of information gathering; inappropriate outcomes; and poor interaction (caller and clinician satisfaction).

The *untimely conclusion* refers to 'jumping out' of the call too quickly or reaching your outcome prematurely. This can happen, for instance, when you think the call will take too long, so there is a great temptation to think, 'Oh well, this is going to take several minutes to go over on the phone, I may as well see them.' Although this can seem practical, if you are not going to devote time to a phone call (and bearing in mind what you are trying to achieve; see section 1.4), there is little point to the phone call in the first place. The default outcome, when trying to deal with calls quickly, is typically seeing the patient. Devoting time to phone calls is an investment. You may reduce other inappropriate contacts or gain greater acceptance of telephone interactions in future.

Time pressures can and do lead to a lack of information gathering. In order to keep the call on track and deal with it 'efficiently', the triager may use closed questions that can result in vital information being missed or not passed on. The triager may 'cut off' callers when they are trying to relay information in order to keep the call moving quickly and this may affect the relationship and 'caller satisfaction' (see section 1.4). When things go wrong in a call, it is often linked to a lack of information gathering on behalf of the triager – 'He didn't tell me that' is not a good enough defence. Your governing body will look at whether you asked enough questions to determine what was relevant and whether you probed sufficiently, given what you were told.

Following on from the previous two points, the natural conclusion will be that there is a risk of reaching an *inappropriate outcome*, either seeing patients who don't need to be seen, or not seeing patients who do need a physical and visual assessment. Either of these outcomes has already been addressed as a risk.

Finally, a *poor interaction* can mean a variety of things, including everything we have already mentioned about outcomes, communication problems leading to caller dissatisfaction and whether clinicians feel that they have done a good job. Clinician satisfaction is equally important – you need to know you have acted appropriately and get job satisfaction. One last risk associated with clinician satisfaction is burnout. Taking call after call after call can lead to GPs and nurses feeling as if they are working in a call centre rather than practising medicine or nursing. When you don't enjoy the task at hand, there is no driver to do it well.

There may well be other risks you can think of when it comes to telephone care, but knowing what the risks are, and how you can avoid or manage them, is the key to successful and safe telephone consulting. Whatever the risks, your role as a clinician is to decide if the risks outweigh the benefits, or if they are too great, in which case the safest option is usually to make sure that the patient is assessed face to face.

Knowing where the risks are is crucial, but what do you really want to achieve from your call?

1.4 What do you want to achieve from a phone call?

Many individuals perform telephone triage without really thinking about what they are aiming to achieve by using the phone to care for patients. They implement telephone consultations for a variety of reasons, some of which we have discussed previously, such as trying to reduce the need to see patients, managing demand or overflow, etc., or just because they think they should be offering telephone access, as it is 'expected' to be part of their service delivery model. A clear vision and understanding of the purpose of the phone call will help you to achieve the right outcome if, for instance, you aren't confident about when or why telephone advice should be given (i.e. providing only self-care management advice). Without this understanding, you may decide to have patients referred to a face-to-face consultation when it isn't necessary. If you continue to lack confidence, and still feel unsure about telephone work despite reading this book and perhaps undertaking additional training, you may not be the right person to carry out telephone triage. Seeing everyone is not the best option for you or your patients, as we have already discussed. If this is happening, you may need to think about whether it's better to empower other staff, such as receptionists or call handlers, to ask a few key questions and arrange an appointment. Having a clinician carry out telephone assessments that are ineffective only wastes time and adds to the workload. Telephone triage is a *clinical skill* and, like any other clinical skill, you can be very good at it or very bad – it's not for everyone.

So what should you be aiming for? I believe that there are three very simple, but absolutely key, principles that you should be aiming for with telephone triage, as summarised below.

---

1   *to determine whether patients need to be seen or their requests or problems can be managed over the phone*
2   *if they do need to be seen, to define when, by whom and where*
3   *to have patients or callers leave the call satisfied with the way you have dealt with them – even, perhaps, 'happy'.*

These principles may seem too simple, but you'd be surprised how often they are not understood or targeted. Other objectives seem to take control and result in a call that is overly long or unsafe. The most common problem that I have encountered is when the clinician is determined to 'diagnose' the problem and focuses on that rather than reaching an outcome as quickly as possible. When it comes to diagnosing, I fully understand and accept that it is an important part of clinical work. However, when it comes to an assessment that doesn't include physical or visual confirmation, diagnosing should be your secondary, not your primary, aim. Each call will require that you have a working or differential diagnosis on which to base your decision making, but *avoid the need to keep asking questions that are all about diagnosing, rather than ending the call when you know what your outcome is going to be.*

Delaying care can cause harm; if spending time confirming what the diagnosis is won't actually change your outcome, *stop* triaging and get the patient seen. For example, if you suspect a deep vein thrombosis or a myocardial infarction from your initial information gathering and from how ill the patient sounds, will any questions about immobility or whether the patient smokes or has hypertension make any difference to your outcome of emergency care? No? So why do you need to know this now? *Get the patient seen* – questions about causes and making an absolute diagnosis can wait until he or she is safe.

The exception to the principle of stopping your questions once you have decided that a patient needs to be seen, is when further questioning will help establish *when* care should be provided, *by whom* and *where*. For example, you may have a patient who definitely requires physical examination, but you are not quite sure if it should be urgent or routine care and so further questioning is about determining the safest time frame in which to get the patient seen. Alternatively, another type of care provider may be best, e.g. nurse versus GP, so further questions will help confirm that, or you may need to ask more questions to make sure that the patient doesn't need secondary, rather than primary, care. Unfortunately, I have heard many calls in which the questions are superfluous to the outcome – it was obvious after the first minute or two what the outcome was going to be, but the call goes on and on. If someone needs care urgently but the clinician keeps asks questions just to determine or confirm the diagnosis, lives can be lost.

Other reasons for calls over-running unnecessarily are when the clinician simply doesn't know how to close a call down, or gets 'hijacked' by the caller who goes on to ask about several matters unrelated to the original request (see Chapter 6); whatever the reason for the call being overly long, patients can be put at risk. Likewise, other patients may have to wait too long to be called back, so keeping the first and second principles of what you are trying to achieve in mind will help to focus the call and ensure that it's as opportune as it needs to be.

What about the last principle, though – *callers should be satisfied at the end of the call*, dare we say even 'happy'. Why is this important? Surely it's about giving people the care they need? Well, if your callers leave the conversation thinking that you didn't listen to them and therefore you didn't really help them, or you failed to provide information in terms they understood, the interaction has been unsuccessful. Your callers may not get what they thought they wanted, but they can still be satisfied with your handling of the call at the end of it. If callers believe that you are truly listening to them and that you have addressed their concerns (real or otherwise), they are more inclined to 'like' you and feel that you have cared for them. If they like you, they will trust you and, if they trust you, they will comply with your advice and cooperate more fully, whether by accepting your outcome or by giving you better quality information.

How do you know if someone is satisfied or happy, though? Many of us will simply ask the question, 'Are you happy with my advice?' or 'Is that OK with you?'. One GP told me that he asked callers at the end of each call, 'Are you happy with my advice?', and he recorded that they were *only* when he suspected they weren't! He felt it was good evidence to have if ever there was a complaint, but I felt that he was practising defensively. Understandable to a degree, but, if he suspected dissatisfaction, shouldn't he have addressed it in the call?

If you suspect that someone isn't happy, what can you do about it? Firstly, as soon as you suspect any dissatisfaction, my advice would be to do something about it. Don't leave it until the conclusion of the call to try to 'fix' things. If you have established the caller's agenda at the beginning of the call (see Chapter 4), it is far easier to try to affiliate your intentions with those of the caller right from the very start, rather than trying to tackle it all at the end.

A typical example would be when callers think that they need antibiotics, but you are sceptical about it from the start. Your clinical findings very early on suggest a viral infection, but then you explain at length (albeit correctly) at the end of the call why antibiotics aren't the right solution. If callers don't like you by that time, perhaps because they don't think you have listened to them, they will be disinclined to believe you. You want callers in the palm of your hand, so that they give you the information you need and then trust your decision making. This will only happen if they are satisfied with your handling of the call from the very beginning.

As I said previously, many complaints are not about the clinical outcome, they are about the way the clinician dealt with the caller. I have heard numerous calls in which I thought patients were put at risk by an inappropriate outcome, but the callers left the phone delighted because they were handled in a way that they responded positively to. In other cases, the clinical outcome was totally appropriate, but the callers left the phone thoroughly aggravated, because they were dealt with brusquely.

Think about what you are aiming to achieve by carrying out a triage on the phone. Do you want to reduce the need for a face-to-face consultation, carry out reviews of long-term conditions or manage workload more effectively, for example? Telephone consultation will help you achieve any or all of these aims if it is carried out successfully by abiding to the three guiding principles, but, whatever the reason for undertaking telephone consultation, make sure that you are clear in your objectives and confident in managing care over the phone.

If you want to try to provide as much telephone advice as possible (when it is safe to do so), is everyone else in your organisation working to the same end? Revisit your team's collective aims on a regular basis, preferably armed with data on the outcomes you reach as evidence of how well you are achieving your aims. Ultimately, it is about getting patients to the right level of care, with the right provider, in the right place, at the right time, but you may need to reconsider whether telephone care is right for you or your organisation if you aren't achieving what you set out to.

References

1. Coleman A. Where do I stand? Legal implications of telephone triage. *Journal of Clinical Nursing* 1997; **6(3)**: 227–31.
2. Fortune T. Telephone triage: an Irish view. *Accident and Emergency Nursing* 2001; **9(3)**:152–6.
3. Soanes C, Hawker S. *Compact Oxford English Dictionary of Current English.* (3rd edn). Oxford: Oxford University Press, 2005.
4. Marsden J. An evaluation of the safety and effectiveness of telephone triage as a method of patient prioritization in an ophthalmic accident and emergency service. *Journal of Advanced Nursing* 2000; **31(2)**: 401–9.
5. Crow RA, Chase D, Lamond D, *et al.* The cognitive component of nursing assessment: an analysis. *Journal of Advanced Nursing* 1995; **22(2)**: 206–12.
6. Leprohon J, Patel V. Decision-making strategies for telephone triage in emergency medical services. *Medical Decision Making* 1995; **15(3)**: 240–53.
7. Tate P. *The Doctor's Communication Handbook.* (6th edn). Oxford: Radcliffe Medical Press, 2010.
8. Campbell JL, Fletcher E, Britten N, *et al.* Telephone triage for management of same-day consultation requests in general practice (the ESTEEM trial): a cluster-randomised controlled trial and cost-consequence analysis. *The Lancet* 2014; **384(9957)**: 1859–68.
9. Huibers L, Smits M, Renaud V, *et al.* Safety of telephone triage in out-of-hours care: a systematic review. *Scandinavian Journal of Primary Health Care* 2011; **29(4)**: 198–209.
10. Lattimer V, George S, Thompson F, *et al.* Safety and effectiveness of nurse telephone consultation in out of hours primary care: randomised controlled trial. *BMJ* 1998; **317(7165)**: 1054–9.
11. Pinnock H, Bawden R, Proctor S, *et al.* Accessibility, acceptability and effectiveness of telephone reviews for asthma in primary care: randomised controlled trial. *BMJ* 2003; **326(7387)**: 477–95.
12. Bunn F, Byrne G, Kendall S. Telephone consultation and triage: effects on health care use and patient satisfaction (Cochrane review). In: *The Cochrane Library*, Issue 3. Chichester: Wiley, 2004.
13. Thompson F, George S, Lattimer V, *et al.* Overnight calls in primary care: randomised controlled trial of management using nurse telephone consultation. *BMJ* 1999; **319(7222)**: 1408.
14. Curtis L, Burns A. *Unit Costs for Health and Social Care 2015.* London: Personal Social Services Research Unit, University of Kent, 2015.
15. Houts PS, Bachrach R, Witmer JT, *et al.* Using pictographs to enhance recall of spoken medical instructions. *Patient Education and Counselling* 1998; **35(2)**: 83–8.

Chapter 2

Communication skills

2.1 Telephone communication skills – are they different from face-to-face communication skills?

Are the communication skills and techniques required for talking on the phone and assessing patients in that way different from the communication skills needed for a face-to-face interaction? Yes, they are, for fairly obvious reasons, but many clinicians make the mistake of underestimating the importance of understanding the differences. It's not simply a case of giving and receiving information, but more about making sure that you have really listened to callers and understood the information they have conveyed.

Even more notably, your ability to communicate on the phone is often dependent on your *relationship with callers.* If they feel listened to, they will like you; if they like you, they will be more inclined to trust you; if they trust you, they are more likely to comply with your advice and decision making. *In short, it is all down to how the caller feels about you.* This is a difficult concept for many of us to grasp initially. The relationship between a patient or carer and the clinician has always been one of trust, but, when it comes to telephone communication, it is harder to develop that trust – especially if the caller is worried that 'you can't diagnose over the phone'. Many patients and carers will have trouble believing that you can care for them when you haven't touched them, looked at something or listened to something. You can face a huge barrier even before you start your assessment. That barrier will only be overcome if you know how to engage in the way the caller needs you to – and therein lies the difficulty. We can misread how callers want us to interact with them in the absence of being able to judge them visually.

The foundation of any telephone interaction is good communication, as we know, but under a very unique set of circumstances, i.e. those of urgency, anxiety, stress, lack of physical examination and sometimes even an absent patient! You may be asked to make judgements about patients' care without having some communication with them directly, through either verbal discussion or physical examination. In telephone triage you may be expected to help patients who are not present at the time of the call and/or with whom you are unable to communicate directly, e.g. if his or her first language is not yours. It is because of these issues that the way you communicate is absolutely vital. Poor communication can lead to mistriage and harm, so what does 'good' telephone communication entail?

An effective dialogue

Good telephone communication means that you will have created an effective dialogue, which simply put, is *an equal exchange of information that makes sense to you and the caller and in terms that you both understand.* This effective dialogue will lead to a more accurate triage and diagnosis, reducing the risk of errors and of missing vital information. It makes sense that if you can't communicate effectively with your caller, the chances of mistriage are considerably increased. There is a lot of evidence available to indicate that, when it comes to risk management of telephone triage, one of the biggest risks, and therefore cause of complaints and untoward incidents, is in relation to communication. Research findings have suggested that communication is a source of clinical risk:[1]

- to patients in terms of clinical outcomes and satisfaction
- to clinicians in terms of their psychological wellbeing or of receiving a complaint or being sued.

Other differences between face-to-face and telephone communication

There are other interesting differences between face-to-face and telephone communication that can influence the interaction.

- *Telephone conversations often use more formal language than face-to-face dialogue.* A number of studies have suggested that, when two parties cannot see each other, the language used sounds more like the language or linguistics that would be associated with written text. This formality can make the interaction seem less personal and, in turn, can affect your relationship with the caller. It is difficult to build a level of trust when you are not connecting on a personal level.

- *You are less likely to reach a compromise through negotiation over the telephone.* Studies have suggested that, when negotiation is required and the parties cannot see each other (and when one party had what it thought was the stronger case), the side with the stronger case often won the negotiation.[2] Conversely, in a face-to-face encounter, both parties were more willing to compromise. Negotiation can also utilise other physical attributes, such as reassuring nods of the head or emphatic shaking of the head. Direct eye contact can convey trust and confidence. When appropriate, physical contact, such as a reassuring hand on the arm, can also convey that you are trying to engage with the other person and that you are 'on their side'. When talking on the phone you don't have any of these tools available to you, which makes negotiation harder. What you do have, though, is your tone of voice, which we will discuss in the next section.

- *The lack of visual input can lead to a lack of social inhibitions that usually temper the conversation.* Not being able to see the other person makes it easier for some people to 'let off steam' or become emotional more quickly. If there are silences on the phone and you have omitted some form of acknowledgement or 'filler' (e.g. mmm, yes, OK, I see, oh dear) to let the caller know that you are listening, the caller may interpret this, as 'you're not listening to me'. In a face-to-face encounter, we can show that we are listening to someone by just looking at them or by inclining our head to show sympathy. As they can see us, they can also tell if we are doing something else, such as reading a computer screen or tidying up the surgery, and we don't have to fill in the silences. On the phone, a silence can be perceived as lack of interest, which can make the caller more emotional when he or she may already be acutely stressed.

- *It's easier to talk over someone on the phone.* When you can see the other person, you are able to see when someone is about to speak, or you can indicate that you would like to speak by raising your hand, or leaning forward showing your intention to interact. On the phone, you don't have these physical prompts and so it is easier to talk over each other. As we know, if you speak over the top of someone too much without either acknowledging it, or correcting your behaviour, the caller may think that you are more interested in talking than listening. This gives rise to irritation, dislike and then distrust. Once this happens, it's more difficult to get the caller to engage with you and the result may be your obtaining less information or a lack of agreement about the outcome.

Demand versus expectation

Central to the skill of communicating effectively on the phone is your ability to accurately understand what the caller's wants and needs are and to provide the right solution and care to satisfy them. We know that this may not always be possible, in which case the ability to make callers understand why you are unable to comply with their request or demand may make the difference between a satisfied caller and an unhappy one. Using adroit communication skills, you might be able to turn a 'demand' into an 'expectation'. For me, a demand suggests that someone is immovable, while an expectation implies that the caller has an idea of what he or she wants but is open to negotiation. In telephone triage, an expectation is much more desirable than working to a demand – especially when it can put the patient or others at risk.

Many of us will capitulate to what callers 'demand' because we don't think that we will be able to change their minds. For example, the caller may insist on (demand) a home visit and the clinician may feel that they have no choice but to comply, fearing a complaint, even when they feel that an appointment at the surgery may have been more appropriate. It can also be tempting to think that it would take too much time to try to negotiate, as the caller has made it very clear that he or she is going to insist on something, such as antibiotics or seeing you, rather than being advised over the phone, so why should you waste your valuable time trying to change that? It is easier to give in to demands and sometimes more efficient, but if you engage with your callers in a way that they respond to, you are more likely to reach a mutually agreed management plan. Your ability to communicate can make all the difference to whether the caller agrees to your suggested outcome, rather than continuing to demand an inappropriate (and costly) visit, inappropriate medication or a face-to-face consultation when it isn't necessary. Patients' 'expectations' can replace patients' demands, and that is what we should aim for in a telephone triage, but how do we do that?

2.2 How do we really communicate?

From a number of studies, it would appear that, in order to communicate, we require a sender of information, a receiver of information, the message itself (the information being exchanged) and the use of differing modes of communication, i.e. the telephone, face-to-face communication, texting, emails, letters, etc. Messages or information sent and received will also go through a form of encryption (coding) and decryption (decoding) between the sender and receiver,[3,4] and this is usually when miscommunication occurs. For communication to be effective, it must be received and understood clearly on both sides. When it comes to telephone triage, information should flow in both directions, otherwise the risk of miscommunication, and then mistriage, is high.

The elements of communication

If we think of communication as a complete entity, there are various elements that are used to communicate, and studies have suggested that, when *thoughts and feelings are involved*, communication consists of body language, tone of voice and words.[5,6]

These findings have often been misinterpreted. It is not always linked with the situation for which it was intended (i.e. when communicating thoughts and feelings) and, as it is not directly associated with a patient–clinician relationship, many of us may not want to accept these findings as being applicable in a healthcare setting. As I have suggested, however, telephone triage is very much about relationship building, which includes your ability to interpret and manage another person's thoughts and feelings. Ultimately, I believe that telephone consultations very much come down to how the caller *feels* about what is happening and how we all *think* that the interaction has gone. As clinicians, we are taught to consider the ideas (thoughts) and concerns (feelings) of our patients, therefore I feel that it is entirely appropriate to use Mehrabian and colleagues' findings[5,6] and apply it to telephone care settings.

Face-to-face communication

When asked where we derive our information from, the three elements reported within a face-to-face communication setting are usually:

1 *body language* and non-verbal communication – such as nodding the head, folding arms, eye contact, facial expressions and anything that we comprehend as a result of what we see
2 *tone of voice* – how we say something, what inferences are used and how we choose to emphasise things
3 *the words* – what we actually say, the information that is passed on verbally.

What proportion of face-to-face communication does each of these elements account for (see Figure 2.1)?

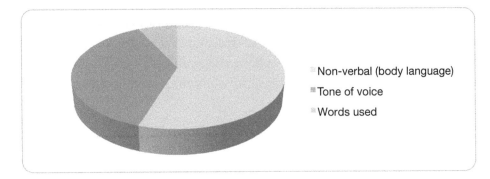

Figure 2.1 Face-to-face communication.

- 55% relates to visual cues, i.e. body language and facial expression.
- 38% relates to the tone or inflection of the voice.
- 7% relates to the actual content of what you say or the words used.

Telephone communication

When it comes to the telephone, you no longer have the body language that previously accounted for 55% of your ability to communicate. As you cannot see the person, and they cannot see you, body language and facial expression are no longer available, but they are replaced by tone of voice and the words used (see Figure 2.2).

As you can see, *84%* of your ability to communicate is now related directly to the tone of your voice and only *16%* comes from the content or the words you use. A lot of your assessment, especially at the beginning, is based on how you think someone sounds, their physical state (breathless, in pain) or how you perceive that they feel about something i.e. anxious, upset, angry, etc. This isn't necessarily expressed verbally, but you pick up this information from how the caller or patient sounds (their tone of voice and other non-verbal clues).

It is difficult to express the importance of tone of voice through written information, as I am attempting to do here, but think about some of the calls you may have taken: how much of your impression of how ill the patient was, or was not, came from the actual information (the words) and how much came from how he or she sounded? How many times have you quoted, 'The parent was really anxious, so I thought I'd better see the child'? Did that decision come from what the parent said or how you thought someone sounded? Even if you are new to telephone triage and haven't yet assessed patients over the phone, think about conversations you have had with other people on the phone. How much of your understanding of the call came from how the

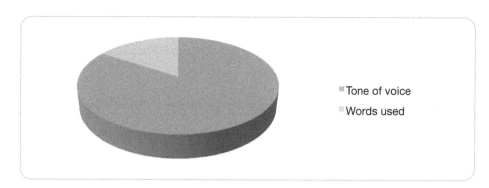

Figure 2.2 Telephone communication.

person sounded, rather than what they actually said? Perhaps you may have spoken to a member of staff at a call centre recently: was your level of satisfaction linked to the information that was given or *how* it was given?

Let us not forget, though, that this exchange is two way. We can use our tone of voice to express our lack of concern as a clinician about what's happening, or our eagerness to end the call, or control it to achieve satisfaction and fulfil our need to make sure that the caller accepts our advice to seek emergency care.

Can you see now that a great deal of the way in which we think about how a call was managed is down to the relationship and how we interacted with the caller, rather than the actual words exchanged?

Telecharisma

When using the telephone, it is critically important to ensure that what you say is clear, but your tone of your voice also has to convey confidence in what you say, your state of mind and attitude. So your first challenge is to develop *telecharisma*! Telecharisma is that personality or character, conveyed through your voice and manner, that lets your callers know that you are interested in them and are there to help them as quickly as you can. Some of us can have a 'telephone voice', one that is reserved for the phone alone, but you also need a telephone personality with which you can engage with your callers almost instantly.

You have to have many 'scripts' when performing telephone triage: scripts that range from how you introduce yourself to giving advice on medication or self-care. The trick to communicating on the phone, however, is never to sound scripted. To all callers it should sound as if this is the first time that you have said something, that you are uniquely interested in them and that this isn't the millionth time you have told patients to drink plenty of fluids when they have a fever. You do this by using the tone of your voice – concentrate on the words alone and you will sound scripted. Once that happens, you can disengage your caller.

So, how do we ensure clear communication?

When it comes to telephone triage, we can never ensure absolutely clear communication, but understanding where the potential for miscommunication lies at least reduces the risk of it happening. One of the biggest problems is when communication becomes one way instead of two way. Typically, one person does all the talking (sending) while the other does all the listening (receiving). This means that you are not necessarily exchanging information in terms that you both understand, as you are not checking your understanding of the other person in the absence of being able to check it visually. Many of us are guilty of doing too much talking and not enough listening on the phone, typically because we think that callers have contacted us for advice, therefore it is up to us to offer that. However, that advice must reflect what callers have asked for, either intentionally or non-verbally – not just what we think they need to hear.

What happens if information flows in only one direction?

To demonstrate a situation in which information flows in one direction only, try the following exercise to see what happens when information in an audio, or 'voice only', form is passed on.

Exercise 2.1

You will need blank pieces of paper (but not pens) and someone else to do this exercise with (or as many people as you like). One person must act as the sender (giving the information) and the other person or people will be the receiver(s) (carrying out the sender's instructions). Once everyone has a piece of paper, the sender must ask the receiver to follow the instructions (see below) and the sender will do exactly the same as the receiver, *but the sender and the receiver must not be able to see what the other is doing*, i.e. the sender should stand behind something or turn their back.

> *Sender: Hold the paper in your hands and follow my instructions:*
> i.   *fold the piece of paper once*
> ii. *tear off a corner (emphasise the word 'a' each time)*
> iii. *fold the piece of paper once*
> iv. *tear off a corner*

  v. fold the piece of paper once
  vi. tear off a corner.

Now ask everyone to unfold their pieces of paper and compare the sender's piece of paper with the receiver's. When the receiver(s) couldn't ask any questions and couldn't see what the sender was doing, did you all arrive at the same outcome, i.e. a piece of paper that looks exactly like the sender's, or does everyone's paper look different? I would guess that there is a high degree of variation between the pieces of paper, but how did it feel when you couldn't see the other person and communication was only one way?

This is actually a very useful way to understand both the concept of 'senders' and 'receivers' and also to see how even a very simple instruction can be interpreted in completely different ways. The emphasis on the word 'a' for instance can be interpreted as tearing off only one corner, but, if the paper has been folded so that the corners are together, receivers can tear off two corners.

Now, on the phone, I know that you aren't going to be folding pieces of paper with your callers, but you often exchange information in one direction only, so how do you know that you have understood each other?

Illustration of one-way communication

A good real-life example of one-way communication often occurs when you give callers instructions on how to take medication, e.g. dosage and frequency. If they don't repeat their understanding to you, how do you know that they will take the right dose at the right time? The only way to make sure is to ask them to accurately repeat your instructions to you. To do this without sounding patronising, or disengaging the caller by intimating that you don't trust them, is quite difficult. I have found that a good way of asking the caller to repeat something to me without doing either of these things is to make it all about my ability to give the information, rather than any mistrust of the callers' understanding.

For example:

> *Would you mind repeating that to me, as I want to make sure that I gave you all the information you need?*

Or

> *That could be quite confusing. Just to make sure that I have been clear, would you mind telling me what I just told you?*

Or

Would you mind repeating that to me to make sure that we both understand what's going to happen?

I have even found it useful sometimes to say outright:

For my own piece of mind, would you mind repeating that back to me as I want to make sure that I was clear.

Can you see that, in each example, I have put the emphasis on my sending the information, or on both of us, rather than sounding as if I'm checking that the callers were receiving it? This method can work in almost any circumstance when you want to check that other people have not only heard what you said, but that they also fully comprehend it.

What happens when information flows two ways, but you can't see each other?

Try the following exercise to see what can happen when information can flow in both directions, but you still can't see each other, as would be the case in a telephone triage.

Exercise 2.2

You will need one other person to do this exercise with you.

You will need 20 building blocks, of which there are ten pairs in different sizes, shapes and colours. The sender and receiver should have ten bricks each, one of each pair, i.e. they should both have the same bricks. Without letting the receiver see, the sender should build a small, but not too simple, model using all 10 bricks. Make sure that the receiver cannot see the completed model. Sit back to back with your partner so that you can't see each other (as in a telephone call) and describe your model to the receiver and ask him or her 'to build *something* that is an exact replica of my model by following my instructions'. It is important that these precise words are used and you reiterate that it must be *something* that's an exact match, if asked, 'Do the colours have to match?'.

Allow only 4 minutes in which to complete the task and, if possible, have a third person tell you both at regular intervals what time has passed or what time is remaining. If you don't have a third person, put a clock somewhere so that you can both see it and make sure that you do not exceed the allotted time.

Now without turning and looking at each other, or seeing what the other person is doing, the receiver should see if he or she can achieve an exact replica of the sender's model. As this is an exercise in two-way communication, though, remember that you should ask each other as many questions as you like but not look at each other until the 4 minutes have passed.

Does the receiver's model look similar to the sender's? How did you feel as you were completing the task? What made the task easier for you and what made it more difficult? Did the time constraint affect you at all and, if so, why?

I would hazard a guess that the models are different, but why is this a good way of demonstrating two-way communication in a telephone triage? Well, using a three-dimensional (3D) complex model represents how difficult it is in telephone consultations: the person on the phone is a complex 3D creature, who may have trouble expressing what's wrong. You have to build a mental image, or model, of what's happening, but did either of you jump into the task without qualifying whether you had to complete the model? Remember, the instructions were to build 'something'; they did not say a 'complete' model. In a telephone triage, it is very easy to jump into the call without correctly establishing what you are going to be assessing (see Chapter 4).

Did you feel under time pressure? That 'ticking clock' is more than likely going to make you want to rush the exercise, or it could make you feel frustrated, but did this come across in your tone of voice? You and your partner should reflect on what happened during the exercise and try to unpick what worked for you, what didn't and why.

During exercise 2.2, how often did you send information and how often did you receive it? Once some instructions had been given, did the person who was building the model (the receiver) tell their partner what it looked like to ensure their understanding of the instructions? If that was happening, you are trying to exchange information, but if the person who was building simply received the instructions and did not pass any information back or ask questions, the exchange is one way and you are more likely to end up with the wrong model.

In any phone consultation, the clinician and the caller should regularly switch from being a receiver to a sender; this means that you are trying to exchange information and it improves the chances of understanding each other correctly. You should ask yourself, 'Did I do all the talking or all the listening, or was it an equal amount of both?' If it was the last and you regularly changed from sender to receiver and back again, that is a two-way exchange of information and automatically a better consultation. Sometimes, though, no matter how hard we try to exchange information, there may be barriers that get in the way. What kind of barriers are there?

2.3 What can be a barrier to effective communication?

There are several things that could affect your ability to communicate on the phone, and the most common is some form of 'barrier', which can originate from you, from the caller, from both or neither. Some of these issues have been covered in the section on risks of triage (see Chapter 1, section 1.3), but it is useful to revisit them here.

- *Poor telephone connection or mobile phone reception.* This can be danger-ous. If you miss words or the caller misses your instructions or questions, you must decide whether to risk disconnecting and ringing the caller back to improve the connection or whether to continue with the call. This will depend on the nature of the call and other circumstances, such as whether or not the caller is alone and vulnerable – is a poor connection better than no connection at all? If the caller isn't at risk, I would suggest that you terminate the call and try again rather than waste valuable time trying to communicate. It will only reduce your confidence, which in turn will affect your decision making.
- *Language differences.* This is probably the most common barrier to communication that we come across, but it can be overcome using an interpreting service or a relative or friend who can communicate in a lan-guage you both understand. If you choose to assess using either of these methods, however, it becomes a third-party call and that can increase the risks of miscommunication rather than reduce them, so that must be borne in mind. If you really can't communicate with the patient in a language you both understand, you may well wonder what is the point of the triage, as you have probably already decided that the caller needs to be seen, but remember the second principle – how quickly and by whom may still need to be defined. It could be useful to at least hear how the patient sounds. I would suggest that you ask the interpreter to ask the patient to come to the phone and say something to you, such as their name and address or date of birth. It really doesn't matter what,

as long as you can hear how the patient sounds, as this may help you to decide whether you should arrange an appointment sooner rather than later. You might want to consider doing that at least before automatically making it a face-to-face appointment.

- *Learning difficulties.* This is often overlooked, or you might not realise that it is an issue until the consultation has progressed and it becomes apparent that the caller is struggling to understand you, or explain things. The level of comprehension of the caller can be a risk, as we discussed in Chapter 1, and poor comprehension can prevent good communication or an accurate exchange of reliable information. Where you suspect that this is the case, it would probably be safer to see the patient.

- *Hearing problems.* Usually associated with the elderly, but not exclusively, hearing difficulties can automatically make a telephone exchange impossible. If the caller is using the TypeTalk service, which allows written exchanges to and from the caller, this removes 84% of your ability to communicate, so you will need to bear that in mind when dealing with potentially ill callers. If you can't hear how they sound, can you accurately understand how ill they are? If you need to shout, as the caller is hard of hearing, both parties' tone of voice has been negatively affected and is therefore less reliable as a means of communication.

- *Speech impediments.* A stutter can make for a prolonged conversation and needs to be handled delicately to avoid talking over or disengaging the caller. It is also likely that a patient with this kind of problem would be reluctant to engage in a telephone conversation, so access to services using this method may not be suitable.

- *Stress.* We have already talked about the effects of stress on the caller or the clinician and how anxiety, time pressures, workload, etc., can cause it. Trying to communicate under stressful conditions has an impact on your ability to relay and understand information, making the consultation potentially dysfunctional. Addressing this as quickly as you can in the interaction could save you a lot of time later. You can manage your own stress to a greater degree, but understanding and acknowledging the stress of your callers may help eliminate some of theirs.

- *Lack of rapport or trust.* We have discussed the importance of your relationship with callers already, but, if callers don't trust you, or you have a poor rapport, communication can be negatively affected. They will be less inclined to give you information and you can end up with a very stilted conversation. Moreover, if you suspect that you are not being given enough information, you will not be confident in your decision making and will probably choose to see patients who may not need to be seen or risk not seeing them when you may have needed to.

- *Missing social cues.* These are the cues that are missing as a result of not being able to see each other, such as politeness or not interrupting. On the phone, a lack of social cues can lead to an impersonal or more formal style of communication and less negotiation.

- *Poor historians.* Sometimes callers cannot provide you with the information you need for your assessment, as they can't recall facts, such as an elderly patient suffering from dementia or in the case of a small child. On other occasions, callers may not be able to provide the history as they weren't present at the time, such as when a mother reports that her child was taken ill at school. As she wasn't with the child, she can't tell you what happened.

- *Third-party calls.* As discussed previously, this is probably one of the riskiest types of call, as the patient is not speaking to you directly and, in some cases, may not even be present at the time of the call. A third party may not have the right information and, as a result, the clinical questions may be answered incorrectly, leading to too high or too low a level of outcome. In some cases, however, the barrier can be removed by simply asking to speak to the patient! Many adults ring on behalf of another adult, who is quite capable of speaking to you, but for whatever reason, has chosen to have someone else talk on their behalf. Just because a third party places the call doesn't mean that the patient will be unable to speak to you.

- *Time constraints.* This was addressed in the Chapter 1, but if the clinician appears 'time driven' and offers few explanations to their callers, making no attempt to build a rapport with them, the risk of communication breakdown is greatly increased. If callers are dissatisfied with the brevity of the call and lack of emotional support, they may fail to follow the advice given, potentially putting themselves at risk.

- *The clinician's own attitude and beliefs.* The clinician may have a degree of bias as a result of his or her own beliefs, whether they are cultural, religious or social. We are all human, and sometimes we may allow our own life experiences to influence our behaviour and become obstacles when it comes to communicating. The 'heart sink' patient, whose very name makes your heart sink, may cause you to listen or communicate less effectively and can affect your attitude. You may have a certain belief or attitude founded on personal experience, such as a complaint or incident, which can cause you to start a call with a predetermined outcome that you strive to achieve, no matter what. You stop listening to any information that could divert from where you are determined to go, and therefore your 'attitude' to a call can become the barrier.

- *Perceptions of patients or their symptoms.* We are all guilty of making assumptions or presumptions about our patients, especially those 'frequent flyers' who call several times a week, but therein is the danger. When we deal with callers who ring about the same, or similar, problems frequently, it is easy to begin your assessment before you even speak to them. You may have decided on the outcome and your treatment based on either prior knowledge of your patient, or based on the information given to you by a receptionist, or other member of staff. When this happens, you are likely to start the call with a closed mind, and you may then miss a vital piece of information that could have changed your advice. Remember the risk of making assumptions in a phone call? This is more prevalent when we are dealing with patients that we are overly familiar with.

How do we overcome those barriers?

Some communication barriers can be overcome with forward planning, such as using interpreters or a third party where there are language or learning difficulties, as mentioned previously, but in many cases the only barrier to exchanging information is a simple lack of attention. If someone isn't listening properly, communication can break down, and either you or the caller may not receive vital information.

Few people are good listeners; listening is different from hearing and it's not easy. When we listen, we don't always hear, and when we hear, we don't always listen. We rarely concentrate hard enough or check that we understand what is being said and we only remember small amounts of information at a time. To listen properly, you need to listen 'actively'.

Active listening

This is a way of listening and responding to another person that improves mutual understanding and focuses the attention on the speaker. Active listening is about 'tuning in' as much as possible by avoiding things that can distract you and prevent you from giving your undivided attention to the caller. Just as importantly, it's about letting the caller know that you are listening. So how do you listen actively?

- *Pay attention.* This is easier said than done sometimes. You must concentrate closely on what other people are saying and let them know that you are listening. Saying 'yes', 'I see', 'OK' or any other 'filler' lets them know that you are still there. They may mention something quite casually that you could miss, unless you are *really* paying attention. If you find your mind wandering during a call, which is not uncommon when you are dealing with lots of calls, you may need to think of strategies to help you focus. Simply being able to stand up while you are talking could help. One surgery I came across installed under-desk cycles to reduce the risks to its team arising from a sedentary setting, and the physical activity also seemed to improve the stamina needed to keep focused for long periods of time. If this is a real problem for you, is it because you really don't like doing telephone triage? A GP told me once that he would often be looking at other things on the internet when he was doing telephone triage. When I asked why he felt he needed to do that, he admitted that he disliked telephone work immensely – perhaps he was self-sabotaging? Although that sort of behaviour can't be condoned, it was a very honest admission on his part, and it shows that telephone work isn't for everyone.

- *Confirm, paraphrase and summarise.* As clinicians, we are taught the importance of regularly confirming, paraphrasing and summarising when taking a history. In telephone work, it is even more important that you do this several times throughout the call, depending on the nature and complexity of the contact and the caller's ability to understand and communicate. I would suggest a minimum of three occasions as an average, but you may need to do it more often if the information is complex, or you feel that you want to take the information on board in small chunks to ensure its accuracy. If callers say something that you feel is important, let them know that you were paying attention by asking, 'So, just to be clear, did I understand you to say …?' or paraphrase what they just said and say it back to them with, 'Are you saying …?' Before you provide the outcome or advice, you should summarise what you have heard and what you have agreed on – bearing in mind that there is no guarantee that the caller is actively listening to you!

- *Picking up on the emotional environment.* Understanding and dealing with any excessive or unusual emotional background shows that you are really listening actively. This may also potentially include the influence of drugs or alcohol, which can affect how people react emotionally. You should consider letting your caller know what you perceive. A good way to tackle this is to use 'I' statements. An 'I' statement is about placing the emphasis on what you perceive, rather than pointing a finger at the caller verbally. For example, '*I* thought I heard some anxiety in your voice', '*I* can hear that you sound somewhat angry about the situation' or 'Am *I* right in thinking that you may have been drinking this evening?'. This is much better than, '*you* sound anxious', '*you* sound angry' or '*you* sound as if you've been drinking'. This allows the caller to either dispel your perception, but not feel as if they are to blame for it, or to acknowledge your perception and hopefully feel pleased that you have been listening to them, thereby furthering their engagement with you.

- *Avoid prejudging the patient, the caller or the symptom pattern.* When you prejudge what is going to be discussed or what you will hear, you will begin to 'jump ahead' and then you are more likely to tune out, as your thought processes become out of sync with the caller or the discussion (see 'Jumping ahead' in the next section for more information). As we have already discussed, prejudging can be dangerous, as you either don't listen to what the caller has told you, or you close your mind down because you want to 'confirm' a judgement/diagnosis you made before you picked up the phone.

- *Beware of 'information overload'.* This expression refers to the fact that we can process only so much information at a time. If too much information is provided, we are unable to assimilate it, and the communication is totally devalued. Therefore, ensure that you provide only an easily digestible amount of information at a time, and check that the caller understands at regular intervals before progressing with the next piece of information, especially if it's complex. If the caller is trying to give you too much information at once, you may need to control the call, so that you can absorb the information at a pace that allows you to understand it thoroughly. When I first began doing telephone triage, I had a terrible habit of trying to give lots and lots of self-care information. I realised after a while that I had completely lost my caller, but I would plough on regardless, just talking more loudly and more quickly to try to regain their attention! I now know that it is better to give small pieces of information and to do it in stages, reassessing regularly whether the caller either wants or needs more, before offering more (see Chapter 4, section 4.5, 'How do you close a call?', for more information).

What can block your ability to listen actively?

The following are some of the things that could stop you listening actively.

1 *Environmental distractions.* For example, busy surgeries, someone waving paperwork in front of you, other phones ringing or other people on phones next to you. It could be the caller's environment that is distracting, such as a loud television in the background or someone else nearby shouting responses. Whatever the distraction is, try to manage it, rather than ignoring it. It will have an impact on your concentration – whether consciously or subconsciously. Ask callers if they would mind turning the television down, as you want to be as safe as possible by making sure that you hear everything they say. Notice I used the word 'safe' rather than 'it would be better'. This often makes callers realise that there is a clinical implication and that you are trying to help them, rather than just irritating them by saying that you can't hear them. They may also think it's all about making it better for you and not them. If the distraction is from someone else in your surgery, I advise a culture of *On the phone, leave them alone.* It can be dangerous to try to get someone's attention when they are on the phone, as valuable information can be lost or misheard. As clinicians, we are also guilty of doing this to other people on the phone, e.g. receptionists. I have seen many instances of GPs or nurses motioning to receptionists that they are going out of the building, or putting something on their desks while motioning to them what they want doing with it. They expect the receptionists not only to understand everything when they are on the phone but also to be able to give their full attention to their callers. This is not possible – please be mindful of distracting others on the phone, especially if they are asking someone what the problem is. They can miss valuable information that you need to be passed to you. I would also recommend that when you are carrying out triage, that you ask other people not to disturb you. Phone work is an audio activity; when someone knocks on your door or 'pops in' between calls, it becomes a visual activity, and your brain then has to return to an audio activity from a visual one and may be slower to respond. This can also be a problem when taking calls in between seeing patients. If you can, try to do one or the other activity rather than both, though I understand that this isn't always possible.

2 *Jumping ahead.* Scientists believe we can think at approximately 500 words a minute, listen at 250 words a minute and speak at about 125 words a minute. Therefore, we can think more than three times as fast

as we can talk, so it is very easy to try to jump ahead and be more efficient, but then you might stop listening while preparing your responses. Doctors are taught to use heuristics, or short cuts, when diagnosing, but, without the visual and physical confirmation, that can be dangerous. Try to stay with your caller rather than moving things along at your pace, otherwise you may miss something.

3   *Mental side trips.* As human beings, we are all susceptible to our minds wandering off during a conversation, usually because something is mentioned that sparks our brains into going off in another direction. For instance, someone might mention neck pain following a car accident and you remember that you have to get your car insurance sorted out – before you know it, that has become your focus rather than the call! Although it is possible to multi-task, or do one job while thinking of another, if you've been thinking about what you're going to order for lunch, what else you have to do that day, who is picking up the kids from school, or how many more calls you have to take while you are taking a call, you may not have listened properly throughout.

4   *Emotional filters.* Is it that heart sink patient calling again? When you are uncomfortable during a call because of something that is particular to you, you can begin to tune out, as it isn't something you are either enjoying or interested in. For instance, you may be uncomfortable listening to alcoholics or people who are drunk, as someone close to you may have been affected by alcoholism personally. The calls are uncomfortable for you and you dislike the situation you are in, therefore you have to be very careful that you aren't 'filtering out' information in order to get the call over and done with. Are you really giving the caller your full attention? Good listeners will avoid allowing emotional filters to unfairly influence the interaction.

5   *Using our 'third ear'.* We are all guilty of using our 'third ear' at times. This is when you might insist that both ears are listening to the patient or caller, but then you catch a fragment of some other conversation around you or you hear your name mentioned. You then begin to participate in another conversation while you are on the phone, albeit discreetly as far as the caller is concerned. If you are listening to something other than your caller, or participating in another activity, are you really listening to your caller or are you tuning out?

Human nature and things outside our control will always mean that we are liable to stop listening actively. *The key, however, is to be aware of when this has happened.* Awareness means that you can decide if you need to ask the caller to repeat something to ensure that you haven't missed vital information. Sometimes it is useful to repeat some of what the caller told you, then ask, 'Did I miss anything?', as a way of trapping any information that you may have missed. Ultimately, you should never be frightened to tell your caller you didn't catch something, as it is the safest thing to do. Another strategy is to say that someone distracted you, or that you dropped your pen, etc. – remember, the callers can't see you, and it would be a reasonable excuse for tuning out!

I hope I have convinced you of the importance of understanding the differences between face-to-face communication and telephone communication. Once you understand the differences and how to manage the restrictions of telephone communication, it will become easier – and you may even improve your face-to-face communications too. Knowing the barriers can help you to manage them, or decide that the barrier can't be overcome and that therefore the safest thing is to see your patient. Sometimes, however, we can be responsible for affecting how a patient communicates with us. For instance, does how we ask a question make a difference?

References

1. Thomas M. *Clinical Risk Management in Primary Care.* Oxford: Radcliffe Publishing, 2005.
2. Morley I, Stephenson G. *The Social Psychology of Bargaining.* London: Allen & Unwin, 1977.
3. Gibson JL, Ivancevich JM, Donnelly JH, *et al. Organizations: Behavior, Structure, and Process.* (14th edn). Boston, MA: McGraw-Hill Irwin, 2012.
4. Kreitner R, Kinicki A. *Organizational Behavior.* (7th edn). Boston, MA: McGraw-Hill Irwin, 2007.
5. Mehrabian A, Wiener, M. Decoding of inconsistent communications. *Journal of Personality and Social Psychology* 1967; **6**: 109–14.
6. Mehrabian A, Ferris SR. Inference of attitudes from nonverbal communication in two channels. *Journal of Consulting Psychology* 1967; **31(3)**: 248–52.

Chapter 3

Questioning techniques

3.1 Is there a right way to ask questions?

Many clinicians tell me that they don't like telephone triage because they get very poor information from the caller on which to base their assessment. I find that a lot of the poor information received is often a result of an inadequate question being asked. A key component of your triage is to have an understanding of the different questioning techniques that may be required at different times within each call. This will ensure that you get relevant and reliable information from which to form a confident, accurate and safe outcome. It is also dependent on your caller's ability to give you the information you require, and this isn't always possible, no matter how many different ways you try asking the same question.

There is no 'one size fits all' when it comes to questioning techniques, and we will cover the differing techniques in the next section, but the way you ask a question is vital. Remember, it is as much about *how* you ask the question, as it is about *what* you actually ask. I hear many calls in which it seems that callers are giving the answers they think the clinician is looking for, rather than a spontaneous response. This is most common with closed questions – but not entirely so. Your tone of voice can convey how you want the caller to respond, as well as the style of questions used. For instance, if you are asking a mother, 'Does your child's sore throat look red if you look inside?', you are likely to get a positive response. If you say, however, 'Their throat doesn't look red does it?', and use your tone to imply that you are expecting a negative response, that is what you are likely to get.

The way you ask the question will directly influence the response you get. Open questions imply that you aren't looking for anything in particular, but you can spend a lot of time trying to get to the point, while closed questions can be leading, and you can end up with information that is totally incorrect or unreliable. Most interactions should use a mixture of open, closed and facilitative questions, except perhaps where a potential emergency is likely (more on this in the next section).

Many nurses employed in telephone triage services are expected to use a clinical decision support system (CDSS), such as NHS 111 in the UK, or other systems that are available from commercial providers (see Chapter 9). These systems are mainly based on closed questions, with a 'Yes' or 'No' response, in order to conduct an algorithmic assessment and arrive at an outcome. The nurse may then agree with this outcome, or may not be able to override it, according to the employer's procedures. The key to these systems, I have found, having used several different ones in my career, is that the user needs to realise that patients are not just two dimensional. The system may require a straightforward 'Yes' or 'No' response, but the patient will often say, 'It's well, sort of …'.

Callers and patients sometimes struggle with a simple positive or negative response, and so the skill of the clinician is in trying to find out the correct information, without leading the caller or being too vague. Occasionally you may need to throw the caller off the scent! By this I mean trying to obtain good-quality information without telling the caller what you are trying to confirm, or rule out, by asking questions in a less direct way. You will then get a more honest answer and therefore one that will mean more to you. For example, if I ask whether the patient is unable to tolerate light, e.g. 'Does the light hurt your eyes?', that's a direct question that can lead the patient into giving a false-positive or false-negative result. If, however, I ask where the patient is and what they were doing (e.g. watching television, at work in front of a PC), or if the curtains are open or lights are on, I can find out if they have photophobia without asking directly. If they respond that they have had to close the curtains, or seem uncomfortable if the lights are switched on, I am more likely to trust that photophobia may be an issue.

The way the question is asked can have a direct bearing on the responses you get. Learning not only what type of question is best but also how to ask the question to ensure that your caller isn't giving you incorrect information is one of the key skills required for telephone consultations. So which technique is best?

3.2 What techniques should you use?

The three most common types of questioning techniques used in telephone interactions are:

1   open questions
2   closed questions
3   facilitative questions.

Most consultations will require a mixture of all three types at some point but, where possible, open and facilitative questions are usually the most effective. However, there are times when closed questions will need to be used as well. A good technique is the 'funnel approach'. This is where you begin with open and/or facilitative questions and then use closed questions to narrow down or confirm the information to reach your outcome (see Figure 3.1).

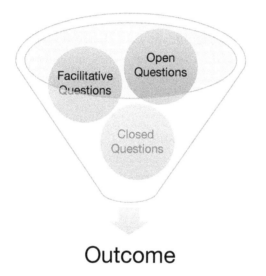

Outcome

Figure 3.1 The funnel technique.

Open questions

A good telephone triage will contain lots of open questions. They allow callers to put things in their own words and you can gain as much information from open questions as you can from closed questions – if you allow your callers enough time to respond. One open question could give you all the responses to several of the closed questions you were about to ask.

Characteristics and advantages of open questions

- They ask callers to think and reflect on the situation. By reflecting on what's happening with the triager, many callers begin to understand what is happening more effectively and can even self-diagnose. They may also realise that there are other, more significant, symptoms that need to be taken into account but that hadn't been their first concern until they were asked what was happening in a general, open way.

- They give callers an opportunity to express their concerns, opinions and feelings. By being given permission to tell you what the problem is in their own words, many callers will let you know what is really bothering them or what they feel should happen. Knowing the caller's agenda can help the triager manage the call effectively to a mutually agreeable outcome (see section 4.3, subsection 'Establish the caller's agenda').

- They help callers to realise the extent of their problem. Once they have told you what's happening, many patients will not only self-diagnose, but they may also tell you what they think needs to happen, or realise that their problem is less significant than they originally thought and that it can be self-managed. Alternatively, they may also realise that this is a more dangerous situation than they thought and so it needs immediate attention.

Disadvantages of open questions

- You hand control of the conversation over to callers. Many clinicians will actively avoid an open question, as they fear handing over control of the call. They are worried that the caller will ramble, or lose track of the point, and therefore waste time. This is certainly true in some cases, but, until you know this for sure, you should attempt to use open questions. One open question, and paying attention to how the patient sounds, could actually save you time, as it could give you all the information you need to reach your outcome.

- You are expected to find a solution to callers' problems! By asking an open question, some callers will feel that now they've told you what the issue is, they've handed it over to you. It's now as much your problem as theirs and it's up to you to sort it out for them.

- It can lead to pauses and a stilted conversation if callers are reluctant to talk. Some callers aren't comfortable with an open question for various reasons. Some simply struggle to think of how to describe something, while others want you to be direct with a closed question, as they aren't sure what you are looking for. In either case, it can lead to a conversation that is very stilted, which affects the interaction and potentially the outcome.

When are you likely to use open questions?

- At the beginning of the conversation.
- To help callers to open up if they seem quiet or reluctant to talk.
- To get callers to feel good about you – it demonstrates that you are concerned about their health problem and therefore they are engaged and more likely to be compliant.

Typical examples of open questions

- Can you tell me about your problem today?
- How can I help you?
- Can you describe the pain for me?
- What does it look like to you?
- What's worrying you exactly?

Closed questions

There are certainly times when closed questions are appropriate, but, unfortunately, many of us will use closed questions at the wrong time, or for the wrong reason. For instance, I often hear closed questions used when triagers are busy or have lots of return calls to make. They believe that the closed questions will get them to the outcome (and the end of the call) far more quickly. However, they can lead your caller, and then lead you, to many false positives and false negatives, which could make the outcome unsafe or inappropriate.

Characteristics and advantages of closed questions

- They require only a yes or no response, or they can be answered with a single word or short phrase.
- They are quick to answer.
- They help you to keep control of the conversation by focusing the caller and gaining specific information quickly.

Disadvantages of closed questions

- They can lead the caller to give a certain response, especially if a question such as 'isn't it ...?' or 'can they ...'? is tagged on. This is perhaps the biggest risk with closed questions.

- They can close down callers, not allowing them to express concerns or opinions. When you allow only a short response, the caller may feel that they can't mention something in case it isn't relevant or important to you, but it could be very important to the caller. It may make a difference to your decision making.

When are you likely to use closed questions?

- When you want to confirm information by paraphrasing and asking for a 'Yes' or 'No' to confirm your understanding.
- When you need to narrow down the information you need by closing down the caller to get only specific information.
- When you need to sum up the conversation by summarising and asking for confirmation of your summation, as mentioned previously in the funnelling technique.
- In an emergency, or when you need to find out facts quickly, as the patient could be put at risk by prolonging your decision making. For instance, in the case of 'chest pain', you should quickly ascertain how ill the patient is, and whether there are red flag symptoms, by using key closed questions. Only when you have determined that the patient is safe should you revert to more open questions.
- When you want to keep control of the conversation. Sometimes, despite your best intentions, your caller may keep wandering off track and you need to step in and take control to make sure that your triage is efficient and effective. The use of closed questions may focus the caller and allow you to manage the call in a timely manner – but be aware of how you may lead the caller.

Some typical examples of closed questions

- Has she been vomiting?
- Does he have a headache?
- Is the pain in your lower back?
- When did it start?

Beware of multiple closed questions

One final word on the use of closed questions: be aware of the risk of asking multiple closed questions in one sentence. For example, 'Have you had any headaches, vomiting or a temperature'? If the caller responds with a single 'Yes' or 'No', is it in response to the headache, the vomiting or the temperature, or all three? If you find yourself asking multiple questions, you will need to break them down into separate questions to make sure that your understanding of each response is correct.

Facilitative questions

The third type of question is facilitative. The easiest way to think of them is as multiple-choice questions that provide options for callers to choose from, or allows them to suggest their own options. Facilitative questions can help find out information, without allowing the caller to 'ramble' (one of the risks of an open question) and without expressly leading (the classic risk of a closed question). Facilitative questions will provide answers to your questions that are more reliable than responses to closed questions, especially if the caller has provided his or her own option rather than selecting one from the options you originally provided. This is also another good way to 'throw the caller off the scent', as we mentioned earlier. By offering differing answers, you will then feel more confident of the response.

When are facilitative questions most commonly used?

- In crisis situations when you need information quickly but don't want to lead the caller.
- When you want to narrow down the information by providing options to help with your understanding.
- When you want to encourage callers to open up but don't want to hand over full control. By providing options, callers may pick one of the options but may also come up with another that you hadn't thought of.

Typical examples of facilitative questions

- Is the blood bright red, brown or dark red?
- Would you describe the pain as constant or coming and going?
- If you run your hand over the rash, is it raised off the skin or is the skin flat?

Notice that in each case there are suggested answers. You can put forward as many options as you like, but be ready for one that you hadn't thought of.

Once you have some information, you will need to decide what you need to ask more about or what you can safely ignore, i.e. when you need not only just to probe but also to pursue. So how do we do this?

3.3 When do you probe and when do you pursue?

During the course of the telephone interaction, you will need to develop the skill of knowing when to probe initially and when to pursue. At the beginning of the call, you will need to probe into what's been happening, a sort of 'big picture' snapshot. Once you have an initial understanding of the situation, you will then need to decide what you should pursue in more detail. You may need to go back to an overall impression of the situation in your summarising. In Chapter 4, we will discuss your approach to taking a call, but, when it comes to history taking, you may be offered information that is irrelevant or, conversely, of particular importance. Your role as a triager is to determine what is useful and when you actively need to try to uncover more evidence. We can often spend time assessing symptoms that aren't relevant to the current triage or be taken off track by the caller (see Chapter 6).

The initial *probing* approach is used when you need to gather chunks of information quickly and in some cases make a decision quickly, e.g. when you are dealing with an emergency. After you have ruled out the need for an emergency response, however, you will need to spend more time getting lots of detailed information (*pursuing*), as would be the case with a vague abdominal pain, for instance. Most triages will use both approaches: gathering significant chunks of information at the beginning to ensure that a high-priority response can be ruled out and then drilling down, by gathering enough detail to ensure that everything is covered, without wasting time on irrelevant information. You will use the various questioning techniques discussed previously in your pursuit of valuable information – but what constitutes 'valuable' information?

Chapter 4

How to take a call

4.1 Is there a right way to take a call?

The objective of every consultation is to gather valuable information and know what to discount as invaluable or irrelevant information. So how do we do this? One of the biggest failings of some triages is a poor call structure and, in particular, a lack of structure when taking the history. As clinicians, we are taught how to gather a history when consulting face to face. For some clinicians, taking a history becomes chaotic when the visual and physical components are removed. In some cases, it seems that questions are virtually plucked out of thin air and there is no methodology, or indeed organisation, in the call. One of the most important things to observe when carrying out telephone triage is to work to a good structure, which will help you to:

- minimise the risk of missing something
- improve the information-gathering process
- think more clearly
- increase your confidence.

A simple configuration to work to is a clear beginning, middle and end – and this isn't meant to be patronising. Some calls will begin like this:

Clinician: What's the problem?
Caller: He (the patient) has a few red spots on his tummy, with small blisters. He's got a temperature and generally he's not very well.
Clinician: It sounds like it could be chicken pox.

This clinician has just offered a diagnosis up front, which should be reserved for the end of the call when drawing up the management plan. By offering this at the beginning, the clinician not only risks the 'confirmation bias' mentioned in Chapter 1 but has also given the caller information that he or she will have logged and absorbed. It would be unusual, but, if you were the clinician, what if, after some more questioning, you change your mind and decide that the rash is atypical or there are other symptoms that don't fit the clinical picture of chicken pox? Or perhaps, half-way through your history taking you say, 'I think we may need to see him' but continue asking questions and then decide at the end that you don't need to see the patient after all? You will sound as if you don't know what you are talking about, and the caller may lose confidence in you. Even if you think half-way through that a patient may need to be seen, try to avoid saying that until the appropriate part of the call. Not only can premature relaying of the outcome result in the caller losing confidence, it can also affect the questions you ask and you can 'pre-judge' what is happening, or what the outcome should be – a risk for both patient and triager.

Calls can be structured using condition-specific telephone triage protocols (see Chapter 9). In the absence of this kind of protocol, however, a very simple generic model can provide the foundation for your triage. This takes the form of the three key stages of a call: the opening (stage 1), the history taking or information gathering (stage 2) and the management plan or closing the call (stage 3). Adhering to these three stages, and in that order, will provide structure to your call.

The triage model or process actually begins before you even pick up the phone, as there are a few basic things you need to do to prepare yourself. It would not be reasonable to expect an actor to perform in a play until he or she had learnt the lines. In the same way, we should never present ourselves to a caller before we have thoroughly prepared for the consultation. So, before you start the triage, you should prepare as follows.

1   Make sure that you have enough time for the triage. Remember how time constraints are one of the biggest barriers to communication – but I understand that this can actually be one of the hardest things to do in the real world. In today's busy practices, making time for a telephone call can be difficult, but refer back to Chapters 1 and 2 and check the risks posed by being under time pressure.

2   Have the patient's notes available when possible and be ready to take your own notes, either on paper or electronically, whichever is easiest for you. We will discuss your documentation in Chapter 7, but, in the initial phase of the call, especially when you are unfamiliar with the patient,

take a minute or so to read the summarised history, medications and last few consultations if these are available to you. If working in an out-of-hours (OOH) service, look out for previous contacts – especially in children. Do you need to review these? Some clinicians feel confident typing up the notes as the caller begins speaking and, as long as this isn't distracting, go ahead. But there is more on this in Chapter 7.

3 Review any notes entered by other staff, such as receptionists, call handlers or other clinicians, but don't rely on them or expect them to be totally accurate. Remember, previous documenters may not have listened actively and their notes may not be a true reflection of the conversation. Also, callers could have given incorrect information, just to get access to the clinician, or perhaps given only an initial description to a non-clinician when there is so much more they want to tell you. By assuming that previous notes are accurate, you could miss important information, or end up assessing something that was only mentioned to gain access but isn't really relevant. A good way to start the conversation is:

I have all the information in front of me that you gave to (the receptionist, the nurse, the doctor), but would you mind telling me everything again in your own words?

Try to avoid telling them what you have in front of you, in case it's inaccurate. If you say to them:

So you told the receptionist that you are worried about …

you may inadvertently say something that wasn't only inaccurate but the complete opposite of what they told someone else. Also, if they were making things up to get access to you, they might 'play along' and, after discussing something that was totally irrelevant for 5 minutes, they might then say,:

While I have you, can I also just ask about …

However, when asking the caller to repeat information, you should also be ready for the response:

Do I have to go through it all again?

I would that suggest you respond with:

If you don't mind. I have all the information you gave to … in front of me, but it would be much safer if I could hear it from you personally.

Notice the word 'safer', not 'better'. The use of this word makes callers realise that there is a clinical connotation to this and they have a responsibility, as do you, to ensure that the call is handled safely. I have found that the word 'better' may be interpreted as 'better for whom?' and less successful in getting callers to cooperate with me. Also, avoid being pressurised into telling them what has been documented previously if you can, or skim over it, indicating that there was more detail but you are withholding it as you prefer a full description from them personally. I have found that most people are more than happy to talk about themselves; the exception is when they have spent a long time telling someone else what was wrong. If you are worried that they may react negatively to your request to tell them once more what the problem is, try to pre-empt it by starting off with the phrases suggested above.

4   Try smiling as you speak. We know that we can hear a smile in someone's voice. Smiling can affect the tone of your voice, making it friendlier and more interested, which is a good way to start a triage. In telephone services such as those in call centres, workers are often taught to 'smile as you dial'! It may sound a bit of a cliché, but smiling can really make a difference to how you sound. A doctor recently told me how he had put this strategy into practice immediately after attending one of my training session 2 years previously. He happily reported that, since smiling as he introduced himself, he noticed that he hadn't had a single aggressive caller. Very powerful. After the initial introduction, however, only smile when it is appropriate – the last thing callers want to hear if they are seriously ill is someone who sounds too happy!

5   Be ready with a verbal handshake – remember telecharisma? The first words from you and the tone of voice used, must replace the smile or physical handshake you would normally use in a face-to-face situation. Your voice must make you appear welcoming, confident and ready to help your caller.

6   Avoid preconceived ideas. To reiterate the importance of avoiding second guessing what the call may be about, or the reaction of the caller: it's very easy to plough straight into the conversation based on your knowledge of the caller, the past history or the notes entered by someone else. You may

take the call in a completely wrong direction based on those preconceived ideas.

4.2 How do you begin a call?

Now that you are ready to begin your triage, how should you start and what is involved in the first stage?

Stage 1 – Opening the call

If you are taking a 'call from cold', in other words the caller comes straight through to you, you should adapt the model accordingly, by leaving out the irrelevant part of the introduction.

The following model, however, is based on the clinician returning a call following a request to call back, or when the clinician is calling as a follow-up to a previous encounter that requires an additional assessment.

When the call is answered, consider whether you need to identify who the caller is *before* you identify yourself

This can be quite a contentious point, as many clinicians will begin the call as follows:

> *Hello, it's the doctor/nurse here, can I speak to …? (asks for patient/caller by name)*

This may seem reasonable, as there is the assumption that the caller has requested, or agreed to, a call-back and left a number for you to do so. Why shouldn't you therefore identify yourself as the clinician up front? Isn't there implied consent? Many professional indemnity advisors are warning clinicians of the dangers of identifying themselves as healthcare providers *before* identifying who they are talking to. They are warning us that, legally, it could be argued that the implied consent does not extend to identifying yourself to whoever answers the phone, namely that you are a clinician wanting to speak to a certain patient or caller, or that you are ringing from the practice or OOH service, and that you are calling because they have asked you to ring them back.

If the receptionist or call handler has asked if it's OK for you to identify yourself as the doctor or nurse (see Chapter 10 on the role of the receptionist) to whoever answers the phone, then go ahead. Alternatively, if the call-back is likely to go through a switchboard and it has been documented that you have permission to say you're a doctor or nurse, then you can do so. In the absence of specific consent, however, you may need to rethink your approach.

If you know your patients very well, or perhaps they are expecting your call at a specific time and you recognise the voice as being the person you need to speak to, it is likely to be totally acceptable that you introduce yourself as soon as you hear, 'Hello'.

However, if you don't know the patients or their social circumstances you could unintentionally breach confidentiality by starting the call by introducing yourself before you have identified who has answered the phone. There are too many cases in which this has ended in a breach of confidentiality and potentially put patients at risk for me to suggest to you that this is an acceptable approach in all calls.

The worst case of this type of breach of confidentiality that I am aware of, in which a doctor identified himself or herself as such as soon as the phone is answered, but *before* establishing the identity of the person who answered the phone, was as follows.

The GP from the OOH service rang the number left by a young female patient. The conversation began:

> *Doctor calling: Hello, it's the doctor here, can I speak to ...? (names the patient)*
> *Person answering: It's her father, what's this about doctor?'*

The GP managed to avoid saying anything about the reason for the call, but he was told that the patient wasn't available. Now, remember that the number given was the one provided by the patient. After the GP discreetly closed the call without offering any information on the reason for it, the father then questioned his daughter about the call. The father and the brother of the patient forced her to tell them why she had contacted the GP. It transpired that she was concerned that she may be pregnant. Unfortunately, the family believed that honour killings were acceptable and the girl was murdered. Although no confidential information was disclosed, the mere act of the GP identifying himself as the doctor (even though he called the number left by the patient) led to a tragic outcome in this case.

In another case a female patient contacted a service, and, when the GP called back, this was the conversation:

> *Doctor: Hello, it's the doctor here. Is that Janice?*
> *Patient: Yes, how long will you be?*

Doctor: I'm sorry Janice I can't do a home visit until I find out what's the problem. How can I help?
Patient: Just beep your horn when you get here.
Doctor: I'm sorry as I said, I need more information before I visit. What's been happening?
Patient: Have you got the right address?

The doctor was about to end the call when she said quickly:

Doctor: Just answer yes or no Janice: are you in danger?
Patient: Yes, that's right.

The patient was in an abusive relationship and had called the GP for help. She had prepared a story for the abusive partner so that, if he checked her phone, she would say that she had been ringing for a taxi, as taxi companies often phone with information about pick-up times. Following the GP's quick thinking, she was able to send help, but, if the partner had answered the phone, I doubt that the GP would have been given access to the patient after her introduction.

These are extreme and rare cases that you will hopefully never encounter. A safer approach to your introduction might be to ask for the caller or patient first in every case and then wait to see what kind of a response you get. Unfortunately, in today's society and culture, many clinicians have found that, if they don't jump in and identify themselves quickly, the caller won't speak to them and assumes that, particularly if the clinician has a foreign accent, the call is from someone trying to sell them something, such as insurance. This is a very sad state of affairs, but in the real world it is not usual, so how can you get around it?

I have found that this works (remember to be careful about your tone of voice; you should sound friendly, not demanding):

Clinician: Can I speak to (names patient/caller) please?
Person answering: Who's calling?
Clinician: (Names the caller/patient) asked me to give them a ring today. Are they available?'
Person answering: But who are you?
Clinician: I am really sorry, I don't mean to sound mysterious, but they have placed a call today and asked for a call-back. Are they available?

Another approach could be:

Clinician: Can I speak to (names patient/caller) please?
Person answering: Who are you?
Clinician: My name is ... (provides name without title of Dr or Nurse). They
asked me to give them a ring today; are they available?

When put in contact with the patient, the clinician responds:

Hello, it's Dr .../ Nurse ... here. How can I help? (establishes professional
title now that the patient is on the line)

We mentioned previously that there are some exceptions to this approach, such as when you know your patients very well and there is no risk involved in saying who you are as soon as the phone is answered, but there also is another set of circumstances in which it is actually safer to ignore this cautious approach. *This is when you are concerned that the patient's life or limb may be at risk.*

If you have information about the patient that indicates a potential emergency situation, such as 'chest pain', 'fitting uncontrollably' or 'not breathing very well', then you should get access to the caller or patient who needs help, as quickly as possible and worry about your introduction later. You can defend your actions on the grounds that the patient was potentially at risk, so you shouldn't mess around – immediate access is required. You can sort out confidentiality issues once you know that the patient is safe.

Many clinicians feel very strongly that this approach, of withholding your identity until you know who you are talking to, is overly cautious and can in fact get in the way of expediting the phone call. It is up to you as an individual autonomous practitioner to decide on what is right for you and your patient. Underpinning this advice is the need to protect confidentiality at all times, so proceed in a way that satisfies this requirement and keeps patients safe. Being efficient isn't always the priority.

If the caller isn't the patient, always ask to speak to the patient –
where it is appropriate to do so and when the patient is present
Triaging through a third party is one of the riskiest things you can do, as discussed in Chapter 1, and yet so many calls are placed by a third party on behalf of someone who is quite capable of talking to you. If the patient is old

enough to talk to you, is comprehensible and is able to come to the phone, you should ask to speak to him or her. If you are facing a barrier such as 'It's OK, they want me to talk to you. I placed the call' or 'They aren't able to come to the phone', you still need to attempt to talk to the patient. In the first example, you might need to say 'Would you mind if I spoke to (the patient) briefly? I can come back to you at any time to get more information, but it's *safer* if I just have a quick word with them'. Once you have the patient, you may be able to complete your assessment with them.

In the second example, you need to find out why the patient can't come to the phone. Is it because the patient is too ill, the phone doesn't reach the patient or the patient isn't even with the caller? If it's the former, you need to find out how ill the patient is. *The effort it takes to just talk on the phone is minimal, so any patients that truly can't manage this need to be seen and probably quickly.* If a patient has to leave the phone after you begin to talk, see if you can get them back. Again, if that's not possible, as the patient is so unwell, getting them seen quickly is probably the safest thing to do.

What if you discover that the patient isn't present, as is the case in the latter example? Alternatively, if the patient is a child and the carer has spent hours trying to get him or her to sleep, would you ask the carer to wake the child to do the assessment? In either case, how reliable can your assessment be if you don't have access to the patient? This is a difficult question, as it really depends on each individual call.

In some cases, you may still want to attempt a triage, as you want to offer some advice, even if limited. In other calls, you may choose to accept that an assessment isn't possible and the safest thing to do is provide advice on who to see and when, based on the information you have. Lastly, you may choose to advise the caller to ring back when the patient is present or awake.

There are few hard and fast rules in telephone triage, as each case has its own merits and dangers. My advice would be to do what you can, but always to make callers aware of your limitations and make sure that they understand that you can't offer a complete assessment if you don't have access to the patient, therefore you are always going to err on the side of caution. In the case of sleeping children, try to at least establish that they are in a 'normal' sleep, i.e. that they can be roused if needed. If the carer refuses to make sure of this, suggest that they will need to bring the child into the surgery or clinic, as this is the only thing you can do, given the lack of accurate information. That is usually enough to gain some cooperation, but not always.

You should clearly state the need to have the patient present and accessible before you commence your triage through a third party. Failure to do so could mean an inaccurate and unsafe outcome, so check that callers accept this risk if they seem to want to force you into advising them without access to the patient, and document your approach carefully.

If you are still unsure of the need to have the patient present, or to try to speak to the patient, revisit Chapter 2 and the issues around communication. Remember the importance of tone of voice (84% of communication)? If you don't speak to patients, you are at risk of missing how they sound, as well as making assumptions and getting misinformation from the caller.

Identify where you are calling from according to locally agreed protocol

Once you know who you are speaking to, let the caller know where you are from, such as the name of the surgery or organisation. Many OOH service providers, for instance, don't like to be referred to as 'the emergency doctor', and many patients have no idea who their OOH service provider is, so, when you give the name of the service, they can become confused. Find out what is preferred where you work, or agree on a way of naming your organisation among the team.

Check the demographics of patients, where appropriate, especially their current location (this may not be their home address or where they phoned from originally) and if they are alone

As a minimum standard, and especially when you don't recognise the voice of your caller, I would suggest that you ask the caller to give you their date of birth (DOB) to ensure that you have the right notes. Even the most efficient and exceptional receptionist or call handler can pick up the wrong notes and, before you know it, you are entering your documentation on the child's notes, who has the same name as the patient. There are also several cases in which test results have been given to the wrong patient, as demographics weren't confirmed. By checking the DOB, you are doing something to ensure data protection. Many OOH service providers have very strict protocols for checking identities of patients that extend beyond DOB, so, again, familiarise yourself with any locally agreed protocols.

If a mobile phone number has been given and you are facing a potential emergency and the patient is alone, it's vital that you check the location of your patient before you ask any other question, as you need to know where to send an ambulance if they collapse.

At this point, I should say that an emergency in primary care, or in most other services, is rare, but you must always be prepared for one. Patients and carers will ring their GPs or OOH services when they are dying and you could take such a call at any time. The problem is that, because we don't take many of these calls, we're often unprepared, or think 'surely it can't be as bad as that or they would have rung 999'. Patients are renowned for contacting their GPs instead of calling 999, for lots of reasons.

There is more to the simple introduction, or opening of the call, than you may have realised. We must always be mindful of confidentiality and data protection and, just as importantly, we need to make sure that we are able to deal with a severely unwell patient as quickly as possible. Once we have moved beyond all of this, however, how do we take a history in the most effective and efficient way?

4.3 How can you gather information quickly and safely?

Once you have established the introduction and are ready to begin your assessment, you need to make sure that you approach it in a structured way and in a time-efficient manner. You may also, where necessary, have a sense of clinical urgency. So how should you take the history?

Stage 2 – History taking and information gathering

As a clinician, you will probably have a system or structure for taking a history when dealing with patients in your clinic or surgery, but we know that assessing patients based on a history taken face to face is completely different from assessing them over the phone. It's not easy to estimate how much pain they are experiencing, as you can't see the physical signs. You can't gauge how any activities of daily living, such as the ability to walk, have been affected. It takes specific, focused questioning (and listening) to gather enough information to accurately evaluate the condition of the patient. Your understanding, or impression, of the descriptors used will influence your advice on the level of care required. The good news is that a face-to-face consultation comes down in most part to the history taking[1] (80%) and this is exactly what you are doing on the phone – taking a history – so be reassured that much of your consultation is exactly the same. However, you may still need to carry out some form of 'physical examination' over the phone – but based on the caller's interpretation rather than your own observations.

So how do you collect a good, clear and accurate history? I would suggest the following:

Start the consultation with an open question

Even if you have prior knowledge of what the call is about, always start with a question that allows callers to give their own description of what their concerns are, such as 'How can I help today?' or 'You rang about your son/daughter/mother/self. What can I do for you?'. Remember to be cautious about starting with 'You rang because your son has a temperature' or 'So your chest is very tight this evening' or 'You wanted to know about swine flu?', as we discussed in section 4.1. Remember too to be ready for 'Do I have to go through it all again?' as debated in section 4.1, point 3, 'Review any notes'.

Allow the caller time to respond

On average, 30 seconds to 1 minute is sufficient time to get a description of the reason for the call. The 'golden minute' rule[1] is invaluable here, but be careful about giving too much time, as you don't want to lose control of the call or begin to 'drift off'. The key is not to interrupt callers and resist the urge to begin your clarification before they have told you what they perceive as the problem. Make sure you are really listening to what they are saying and focus on that and not on the questions you need to ask just yet. As Steven Covey said 'Most people do not listen with the intent to understand; they listen with the intent to reply'.[2] Pay close attention to the descriptors used. Few patients call their pain 'severe'; they tend to use words such as 'really bad' or 'crippling' or 'terrible'. The way they express the problem will give you an insight into how they feel about it and what their concerns are. You may also find that patients who are known for abusing services will use terminology that they have heard clinicians use – they learn trigger words and phrases to get what they want. Be wary of falling for these tactics. Does the descriptor used match what you are hearing? If a patient is in severe pain, can you hear it in their voice? If a patient is 'struggling to breathe' are they talking to you normally, i.e. in full sentences, or even talking over the top of you! If callers seems to be going off at a tangent, or taking too long to get to the crux of the problem, you may need to intervene by politely asking them to clarify something, or focus them by saying, 'So what's changed to make you ring today?'.

Once you have the caller's description, repeat to them your understanding of the reason for their call

As clinicians we are taught to confirm, paraphrase and summarise the history given to us. This is never more important than in telephone triage, as you can't confirm or rule out anything visually or physically. In one study, patients and clinicians saw the reason for calling differently in one-third of calls in which they both participated. You can easily begin to triage the wrong thing by misunderstanding the reason for the initial call. Remember the brick-building exercise in Chapter 2? If you assume that you have the right bricks, but in fact you haven't, you won't be able to build the right model, no matter how hard you try. I would suggest that you continue to paraphrase and check your understanding at least three times during most triages. If the call is long and complex, you may need to do this several more times, but it is essential that you keep checking that your understanding matches that of the caller.

Establish the caller's agenda

One of the most important things to establish at the beginning of the call is what the caller wants to happen and whether you are dealing with a demand or an expectation, as we discussed in section 2.1. The best way to do this is to ask a question such as:

What was it you were hoping I'd be able to do for you today?

or

Was there anything in particular you were concerned or worried about?

or perhaps

Was there anything you had in mind that you might need in particular?

By finding out what the caller's ideas, concerns and expectations are at the very beginning, you may save yourself some time, as well as learning what you might need to focus on to win their trust. Be prepared, though, for all responses, such as 'I want a home visit' or 'I think I might need antibiotics' and even 'I have no idea, that's why I rang you!'. If it's the latter, I would say, 'OK, that's fine, we are both going into this then with an open mind.' If you clearly establish what the caller is most worried about or if they are the 'immovable object', you have a better understanding of what the call will be like and can take control accordingly.

Think about speaking to children on the phone

As we have established, it's important that you try to speak to the patient wherever possible and appropriate. This may extend to children. The caveat here is that you probably shouldn't carry out a full assessment through the child – that should be done with the carer. However, a brief chat with the child could help you enormously with your decision making. So let's look at the value of speaking to a child and perhaps some rules of thumb you might like to consider.

For example, if a 9-year-old child is brought into the surgery to see you, do you ignore him or her? Do you talk only to the carer? Of course you wouldn't, so why not consider doing on the phone what you would do in a face-to-face consultation, which is usually an introduction or a greeting and a general 'How are you?', 'What's been happening?' or 'How are you feeling?'. When you hear how the child sounds, you begin to get a better understanding of how the symptoms are affecting them and what their general condition is like. If you've forgotten to ask if the child is there, this will also prompt you. If the child sounds very ill, very upset, coughing all the time, thick throated or absolutely fine, you will be able to reach your outcome more confidently and efficiently. You might not even need to ask too many more questions after you hear how the child sounds. If, however, the carer says that the child is outside playing and doesn't want to come to the phone, you may be less convinced about the need to see the 'unwell' child.

A good rule of thumb is to try and routinely ask to speak to children over 8 years old. You have to have the carer's permission, though, to speak to a child, and many will be wary of you asking this, so it takes some delicate handling. You don't want the carer to think that you don't trust them, or that you have an ulterior motive for speaking to the child, so I would say:

> *Would you mind if I said a quick hello to (name the child) and introduced myself? If you were here in the clinic, I would say 'Hello' to them normally and I think it's really important that they know who I am and that we are talking about them. I am going to ask you to tell me all about what's been happening with (name the child again) and we'll discuss what is the best thing to do, but a very quick 'Hello' would be useful. Is that OK with you?*

If you don't get access to the child, I would be very concerned about why not. If the child is under 8 years old, try to decide if it's still worthwhile attempting to speak to the child by considering how articulate the carer is. I have known 2-year-olds who are able to have a full conversation on the phone, while many 13-year-olds will only grunt!

One final point, just to reiterate, is to remind you that you are not going to take the full history from the child, or do the assessment through the child.

You just want to get a brief impression of how they sound to help you with your decision making.

I once asked to speak to a 6-year-old, who, according to her mother, 'needed antibiotics for her tonsillitis'. After asking to say 'Hello' to the child, as discussed, and being given permission to do so, I asked the child where she was as we were talking (I just wanted to hear her talk and thought this would be a good question to lead to other things). She answered, 'Pizza Hut' (other pizza companies are available!). I asked if she had eaten any pizza, to which she responded 'Yes, three bites'. When I then spoke to her mother I said, 'As you probably heard, she told me she was in Pizza Hut, that's excellent news. She also said she has had some pizza to eat, that's really reassuring. Now let me ask you some more questions.' I avoided the need for a face-to-face consultation, as well as antibiotics, because I was able to use the information positively and reinforce with the mother that antibiotics weren't needed at that time. I was also able to tell the mother that the case of potential tonsillitis had been recorded if she needed to be referred, which the mother was hoping for. She didn't call back.

So, just to summarise this point, consider speaking to children briefly to gain a better impression of how ill they sound, but remember that you are still going to take the full history from the carer. If the carer doesn't give you access to the child, why?

Once you are sure you are on the 'same page' as the caller, you need to get a more detailed history, but first eliminate basic red flags quickly

Asking about airways, breathing and colour (ABCs) up front, in almost every call, can reduce the risk of your forgetting to do so when you need to, or asking too late – especially with third-party calls. You may need to use closed questions in an emergency situation. 'It is easier to identify an emergency than rule one out'.[3]

Once you are sure that the patient is not in immediate risk from compromised ABCs, you need to move on to your structured assessment. There are books available on telephone triage protocols that are condition-specific protocols for assessing adults. However, in the absence of a specific triage protocol, one way to take a structured history is by collecting information on the symptoms first, followed by a history of the patient. Without being too prescriptive, this is a generic protocol that can be applied to most calls. You may prefer to take the history the other way round, i.e. patient history before symptom history, or to mix and match, according to the call you are dealing with. As long as you have a structure that you're comfortable with and use consistently, the order doesn't matter. Just be careful of the bias we mentioned earlier, how you can jump to conclusions or assumptions about the patient, or the symptoms, based on prior knowledge. You don't need to complete all of the history-gathering protocol, only as much as you need to, given the urgency of the situation. Avoid becoming that 'system operator' or relying too much on the protocol (see Chapter 9). Use your clinical judgement on each call on whether you gather every piece of information, or if you can decide that you have sufficient information to reach your outcome without going through the whole history.

Three important questions
Before taking a full history, you may find the following three questions invaluable:

1 Where is the patient?
2 What is the patient doing?
3 How does the patient seem to a third party?

Let's look at these in more detail.

Whether you are speaking directly to the patient or to a third party, try to find out *where the patient is*. If you forgot to check that the patient was present in the first instance when the call was placed by a third party, this will help as a prompt. If the patient is an adult and tells you that they are at work, you might begin to think 'Well, it can't be that bad, if you are still at work, but, by then asking, 'What are you doing now at work' or 'What is your job?', you might discover that the caller can carry out their usual tasks. Again, this will help you to determine how the symptoms are affecting the patient and, even if you decide they need to be seen, it may not be urgent. However, if the patient has had to come home from work as they can no longer carry out their job, it helps you to determine that their illness is having a more significant effect on them. It still may not be serious, but at least we know that it has affected their activities of daily living. If the patient is a child, by asking where they are and *what are they doing*, you may find out that they are outside playing or asleep. Whatever they are doing, it can either allay some of your concerns or act as a prompt to find out more about their general condition before going into specific details about what is wrong.

If there is a third party present, even though you should always speak directly to the patient where possible, it might still be useful to ask the third party a general question along the lines of 'How does (the patient) seem to you?'. Remember, don't lead them by saying, 'Do they look pale/ill to you?'. The third party may reassure you by saying something like, 'I've seen them a lot worse than this!'. Alternatively, if the third party says, 'I've never seen them like this before', you will already be more concerned and may not need much more information. If the patient is a child, it may be useful to say to the carer, 'You know (child's name) best. Is there anything in particular that you've noticed is unusual?'.

We are trying to find out not only what symptoms the patient has but also how badly the symptoms are affecting them. Even if you have decided to see the patient, these three questions can help you decide how urgently they should be seen.

Symptom history

What is the chief complaint?

Some patients have multiple symptoms and you need to decide which is the chief complaint, or what you want to assess first. Asking callers what worries them most is useful, but your role as a clinician is to identify the chief complaint, as the caller may not realise that certain symptoms are more concerning than others. For instance, a patient may be suffering from vomiting and diarrhoea but vomiting can be caused by many things and may indicate a serious incident, whereas diarrhoea, is less likely to suggest a life-threatening condition. The patient may feel that the diarrhoea is the most unpleasant, however, so from their point of view that may be the chief complaint. Once you have assessed the chief complaint, if you decide that a face-to-face outcome is required, you may not need to assess any other symptoms over the phone. However, if assessing other symptoms could affect the urgency of your outcome, it may be useful to carry out a secondary assessment.

What are the associated symptoms?

What else is going on? What other symptoms are there? Do you need to rethink the chief complaint? This is the first opportunity to make sure that you have a round-up of all the symptoms as the caller perceives them, but you may need to double-check that they haven't missed anything. For example, if you are concerned about meningitis in a child, the parent may have said that they hadn't noticed a rash, but where did they check and when? Be careful of closed questions, as they can give false positives. General open questions to begin probing about what is happening are best at this point, but, if it is a potential emergency, then closed questions are a priority.

What are the features or physiognomies of the symptoms?
When looking at the symptoms, you will need to consider such things as what type of pain is it, i.e. dull, sharp, constant or intermittent? Does it move or radiate, or is it stationary? If a rash is present, what does it look and feel like? If a temperature is present, how has it been measured (if at all) and what is the reading, when was it last taken, has it increased/decreased? Sometimes, it may help to summarise the symptoms as mild, moderate or severe. If they are leaning towards severe, you are likely to want to have the patient seen, in which case the second principle of how soon and by whom is all you need to decide. Your questioning should be restricted to determining which option is best, rather than further questioning on the symptoms or past medical history (PMH), unless *this will affect your outcome.*

When did the symptoms start?
If this is the first 'episode', when did it start, but, if it's not the first episode, when did the latest and first episode begin? You're not asking how long the symptoms have lasted but rather when they began. If there are multiple symptoms, clarify when each symptom began or became present. Have the symptoms changed in any way or are they episodic or ongoing, i.e. has the patient's temperature increased or decreased? Patients will often contact you when things are getting better! Many patients are looking only for reassurance (50%),[4] and so, when they ring, they will report an improving clinical picture, rather than a worsening one.

How long have the symptoms been present or what is their duration?
If this is the first 'episode', how long have the symptoms been present? If it's not the first episode, how long did the other episodes last? Have they changed in duration? Are they shorter or longer? A change in pattern is significant as it can indicate either a worsening or an improving situation. Again, what made the caller ring at that moment in time if this has been ongoing for some time, either constantly or episodically? Be on the lookout for anything uncharacteristic or atypical of what you would normally expect to hear, given the nature of the call and your knowledge of the patient. Does the pain last for much longer periods of time, or have some symptoms gone, while others have just begun?

What is the location of the problem?

Finding out the exact location of the pain or rash is one of the hardest things to do over the phone and often leads to assumptions or a misunderstanding, due to a lack of clarity. Use terms the caller understands to identify parts of the body, or the size of something, e.g. the size of a 5p or 50p coin. You need to build a mental picture of the problem and be very clear about where it is. Remember the exercise in which you had to draw or build something, but couldn't see it? Treat this mental picture in the same way. Find a point of reference (and possibly use this point in relation to another) to get a clear description of where something is. Never take the caller's own description as being accurate – 'kidney pain' is notoriously misrepresented! You need to build your own understanding of where something is. Lay terms are always best. If you are worried about insulting the intelligence of the caller, don't be. What's better – you obtaining an accurate history, or assuming that the patient knows where their stomach pain is, when in fact it's chest pain?

- Here's an example of using reference points:

  If you put your hand over your tummy button, is your pain above your hand, below your hand or directly under your hand? (Now, let's assume that the answer is above their hand.)

  Keeping your hand over your tummy button (the caller shouldn't move from this point of reference), is the pain closer to your hand, or closer to the bone that runs between your breasts/down the centre of your chest?

  OR

  If you drew an imaginary line around your waist, is the pain in your back above or below that line? (If the caller answers below ...)

  If you drew another line where the cheeks of your bottom meet your thighs, is the pain closer to your waist line or the one on your thighs?

- Can you see how using points of reference can help you build a much clearer picture of where something is? Don't skip over this part of your assessment – it's vital that you have a good, clear understanding of the location of something, otherwise you may get a completely wrong impression, which could have serious consequences.

Does anything make it feel better or make it worse?

- Has the patient tried something to make them feel better, or improve the symptoms? Did it work? This includes anything from medication, to holistic approaches, ice packs, warm packs and even positioning. Do certain positions aggravate or help? Can you get patients or relatives to do some of the physical examination for you? For example, getting them to put their chin to their chest to check for neck stiffness, pressing on their abdomen where it's painful to see if it's made worse by pressure, or does standing up make the patient more dizzy than before. You need accurate and up-to-date information on what makes things better or worse. If they haven't tried anything at all yet, you have a better idea of what you can offer by way of self-care. But if they have exhausted all of the usual self-care methods, you may decide that they need to be seen.
- Checking on medications tried. When it comes to finding out which medications have been tried, you need to be very clear on what they have taken. This is often one of the things that's assumed in a call – that patients have taken the proper dose. There are five parts to this subject:

  1 What have they taken?
  2 How much have they taken (dosage)?
  3 When did they take it and how much *that day*?
  4 When did they take it and how much *if the symptoms have been present for more than that day*?
  5 Did it help?

Again, never assume anything when it comes to medication. I have known some patients (forgive me for saying so, but it seems to be particularly men) insist that they've taken pain relief, but, on further questioning, it transpires that they've taken 500 mg of paracetamol, once, the day before and for a pain that has been going on for 3 days – and then they're surprised when it didn't seem to help! Parents will often tell you that they have given the child a 'teaspoon of paracetamol'. On probing, they will then clarify that they used a household teaspoon (which typically contains perhaps 3 mL and not the 5 mL you might have expected) and that the dosage on the bottle was for a younger child. So, in fact the child has had only one-quarter of the dose they could have had. Conversely, they may have chosen to avoid giving any pain relief, as they were worried 'you wouldn't see how ill they were' or that 'it would mask meningitis symptoms'. Finding out exactly what has been given is crucial to your management and advice and is often done poorly in an assessment (see Chapter 6). Do you have any medication left to suggest? If not, how quickly do you need to get the patient seen, or can you prescribe additional medication and still treat at home?

Having gained the information on the symptoms, other factors may need to be taken into consideration about the individual patient.

Patient history
Now we need to find out more about the patient and relate that information to the symptoms, if necessary. So let's approach this in a structured way too. Once again, though, you may choose to ask these questions in any order, and some may not be relevant for each triage call, so you will need to judge within each call what you require.

What is the patient's past medical history?
What is relevant to the assessment? Many clinicians working in OOH services feel vulnerable when they may not have access to the patient's medical history (although this is becoming less common with system integration). I have found, however, that having access could be both a blessing and a hindrance. You may become a better triager when you learn not to rely on the system to tell you what has happened previously. If it was relevant to the situation that day, you should have been double-checking the history anyway. Having said that, some patients are so poor at being able to give a significant history (or insisting that there wasn't any when they were on a huge list of medications) that having access to the history is invaluable. In most cases, you don't need a full history, as it is more about what's happening that day, but think about anything that may be a contributing factor to their current state. For instance, if they have abdominal pain, have they had surgery? If there's chest pain, is there a history of hypertension? You need information to help with your differential diagnosis, but, unless it's relevant to the immediate handling of the situation, ensure that patients are safe first, before getting caught up in pursuing all of the medical history. I have heard some calls that have been unsafe, as the clinician spent too much time finding out about previous history when the patient needed urgent attention.

Are there any particular risk factors for this patient?
Any long-term conditions such as diabetes or chronic obstructive pulmonary disease (COPD) need to be considered, but be careful of associating any

problem with these conditions before completing your overall assessment. Don't get hung up on things such as blood sugar readings or insulin dosages, unless you think it is relevant to the current problem and your management of it. If the patient is ill, sounds lethargic or incomprehensible and he or she has diabetes, would knowing what the blood sugar level is make a difference to your outcome? Are you trying to reach a diagnosis? You are more likely to need to suggest urgent transfer to hospital, depending on the history, regardless of what the blood sugar level is. Remember the first and second principles of telephone triage – once you decide that someone needs to be seen, any additional questions should relate to by whom and when.

If a patient has pain and swelling in their calf, sounds breathless and complains of pain in their chest, do you really need to know if they have travelled recently or been immobilised? In a similar way to the previous point on PMH, make sure that your questions about any potential risk factors are appropriate, *given the clinical situation at the time of the call.* Is the patient safe first and foremost? I understand that knowing about potential risk factors can help with the diagnosis, but the priority is to determine what care needs to be given first and in the case of a calf pain with other associated symptoms of a deep vein thrombosis (DVT) or pulmonary embolism (PE), knowing about recent travel won't affect your outcome.

Does the patient's age increase the risk?
Sometimes the biggest risk factor that you need to consider is simply the age of the patients. They may be too old or too young to take the risk of giving telephone advice. Both of these patient groups can deteriorate quickly, but children can also recover very quickly, so there is still a need for the triage.

If you feel that you need to see every child (many clinicians have a lower threshold for children), consider the point of the triage. If you feel that there is little need for the phone call, as you will always choose to see the very old or very young, don't forget about the second principle – namely when and by whom. The triage could still ensure that patients are seen in the right place and at the right time. You may decide that someone needs emergency care rather than primary care after your phone call. Not all neonates are ill – it could be a minor problem, such as a dry patch of skin on the leg that the parent has just noticed, so a phone call could save you and the carer an appointment.

The three 'I's' – recent injury, illness or ingestion

Sometimes symptoms are not immediately associated with a recent injury, illness or ingestion. Vomiting can be the result of a head injury, for instance, but if vomiting wasn't a major issue at the time of the injury, callers may forget to tell you about the trauma until asked. Again, many children suffer from vomiting, but if the carer didn't witness the child swallowing something, they may not offer this as a potential cause, until questioned. Some conditions are a result of a previous infection, such as Guillain–Barré syndrome or hip pain or limping in what appears to be a well child at the time of the call (post-viral hip syndrome). You may need to probe a little outside the box to ensure that the problem isn't related to a less typical cause.

Pregnancy

Any abdominal pain in women of child-bearing age, or any other issues that suggest a potential pregnancy, requires you to ask about the last menstrual period and, just as importantly, was it normal for them? The latter question is often omitted, but a change in menstrual cycles, such as a shorter or longer period than usual, may be important to your working diagnosis. You need to be as sure as you can be that a pregnancy is not possible, before you discount it. Sometimes questions about sexual activity, contraceptive methods and whether a woman thinks she could be pregnant or not are redundant to a certain extent. Teenage girls may say that they are not sexually active over the phone, as a parent may be listening. Women insist that they couldn't be pregnant because their partner has been away, they are on contraception, or their partner has had a vasectomy, and, in all cases, it has still resulted in a pregnancy. (I recollect one call in which a woman insisted that she could not be pregnant, as her husband had just returned from 6 months' deployment in the army and yet she was 3 months pregnant – that was not a pleasant situation for anyone.) If you are concerned that pregnancy may be an issue, it's better to treat each case individually and rule it out by accurate testing, rather than rely on women's own assessments' of whether they could be pregnant or not.

Medications and over-the-counter remedies

The elderly are particularly susceptible to adverse effects from medications, as they are often taking a large amount and various types of medication prescribed by different clinicians. This can cause interactions, which in turn are the cause their illness. Sometimes, it's something that has been bought 'over the counter' that is the cause, e.g. a 'herbal' remedy that is contraindicated with prescribed medication. Other patients may have tried someone else's medication to see how it worked for them and that again is the reason for their illness.

Allergies

Checking on potential allergies should always be part of any assessment but, in particular, where there is swelling of the face, breathing difficulties or where a rash is present. If you are advising or prescribing medication, you should always make sure that patients are able to tolerate the medication and let them know how to check for any allergic reactions if they've never taken it before.

I was contacted once by a GP who had been criticised by the OOH service he worked for because he didn't ask about allergies in a telephone triage case of a child with tonsillitis. He referred the child to be seen (by another GP), who then prescribed medication, but again who did not check on allergies. It transpired that the child was allergic to the antibiotics. I felt that the service was being overly harsh on the triaging clinician, as he didn't prescribe or advise any medication and that the fault was with the prescribing GP, who failed to check it. Having said that, it is good practice to check for any allergies during your assessment, especially to completely rule it out as the cause of some symptoms. It may also be expected of you by the service you are working for, so it is best to find out if this should be a routine question in every case.

Social history

This point should be left almost to the end of your assessment, as it could be a social situation that tips the balance between seeing a patient or not. When looking at the patient as a whole, it can be the social circumstances that make it unsafe to give self-care. For instance, for elderly patients who live by themselves, or in a situation where a child is not acutely unwell, but the carer doesn't seem capable of looking after him or her, you may want to arrange a face-to-face consultation. Home visits often take place because there are several other children in the household who have to be cared for and bringing them all to the clinic in the middle of the night is not acceptable, or appropriate. You may choose to see elderly patients in their home, or with their carers, to see how they are coping. In the case of children who are 'at risk', i.e. they have potentially been neglected or abused, their clinical condition at the time of the call may not sound concerning but, because of the social circumstances, it may be safer to see them physically. If, however, the child is with a foster carer whom you know and trust, the child is then like every other child and not necessarily 'at risk' at the time of the call.

Number of contacts

The number of contacts a patient has with services can in itself be a significant red flag, but it's not so much about the number of contacts but rather:

- the number of contacts, then
- about what, then
- over what period of time.

Frequent contacts about the same problem, over a short period of time, sends a completely different signal from frequent contacts about different problems over a short period of time. Then again several contacts about lots of different things over several months doesn't necessarily indicate any risk. Conversely, if you have a patient that has not been seen in surgery for several years, they may be at higher risk than a 'frequent flyer', as the former rarely seeks care.

Unfortunately, there have been several cases in which the number of contacts has been a huge red flag, but was not recognised as such. In England, the death of a patient in 2005 named Penny Campbell followed eight contacts to an OOH service, of which only the first and last resulted in a face-to-face assessment. This tragic case was the catalyst for significant changes being introduced to the recording and sharing of information in these services. One of the main learning points, I feel, was that there were frequent contacts with non-improving, worsening or changing symptoms in a patient who had previously been in good health. The clinicians involved in the case cited the fact that, as they had been unable to access the record after each consultation, they were unaware of the worsening situation. But, even without having this access, or the ability to review the complete health record, the fact that there had been so many contacts, and in such a short space of time, should have warranted a much earlier and complete physical review, in my opinion.

Lastly, many clinicians will ensure that a patient is seen if contact has been made more than twice about the same problem. This is entirely reasonable, but a third telephone call initially may still ensure that the patient is seen at the right time and in the right place – just in case you were thinking, 'What's the point of the third triage then?'

So now we have covered how to take a history in a structured way and to ensure that you capture as much information as you can (given the absence of physical examination), I hope that you are able to understand how risky it can be to rush this part of the call. Your challenge is to get good-quality information, as quickly as you can, and also to decide if you have enough. However, how do you decide when you can stop asking questions?

4.4 How do you know when to stop asking questions?

One of the problems, or risks, with telephone consultations is that the call can go on for too long – a risk if it should have been dealt with urgently and a risk if other patients are still waiting for a call-back. Too much information can also prevent you from thinking clearly: it's easier to become confused or unsure when faced with too much. So how do you know when you have enough information to make a safe decision?

I would suggest that, having taken the history in the way we discussed in the last section, along with an assessment of how the patient sounds, you should very quickly have identified if there is a need for immediate action and should reach your outcome within minutes (sometimes even seconds). If there is no immediate danger to the patient and you are able to take a more complete history (see section 4.3), be prepared to stop at any time when you feel you should act. If you have continually confirmed your understanding throughout the call and it's appropriate to take a full history, take one last opportunity to check that your understanding of the problem still matches that of the caller before you offer advice. You may need to take a moment to reflect on everything before you discuss the appropriate outcome. It's common for triagers to rush into this part of the call, when it is important that you are clear on what you have been told and satisfied that you don't need any further clarification.

You might say something like this:

I just want to pull our conversation together to make sure we have everything we need, before we decide on what's best for you. I am going to go quiet for a few seconds while I go through it all in my head.

Or, perhaps more simply:

Just give me a second while I think through everything.

Then do exactly that. Give yourself some thinking time (hopefully you will find that the caller will take the hint to be quiet as well!) and reflect on all the information to decide if you have everything you need for your decision making. If you have kept to the structure suggested, you should find it much easier to decide that you have completed your assessment and can confidently offer advice.

If you feel that you still need more information, consider how relevant it is. Avoid being sidetracked by irrelevant information, or something totally unrelated to the current situation (see Chapter 6).

I would strongly advise you against offering the outcome and then asking more questions, unless it's absolutely vital. You may become confused and less confident and so might your caller. If, however, you are sure that one more question could alter your decision making to a higher level of safety, you should ask it.

The better you become in your ability to make your decisions quickly and with confidence, the less you will find that you are tempted to ask questions after discussing the outcome. So once you have completed your questioning, how should you now bring the call to a close?

4.5 How do you close a call?

Closing a call is one of the hardest parts of most triages and one aspect that many clinicians struggle with. There are two parts to closing the call: reaching the end of the consultation clinically (including safety netting) and then actually saying goodbye! Let's look at the former first, as this is the final stage of the clinical interaction, then we'll look at how to put the phone down once you know you can't do any more.

Safety netting is of course part of the closing of the call, but as it is also possibly the most important part of any call, it's better to deal with this as a stand-alone topic (see section 4.6). We will examine what can happen when your advice is not accepted in Chapter 5.

Stage 3 – Closing the call

You are now at the point when you are able to offer your advice/recommendation/outcome, but should you consider asking the caller, 'Is there is anything else you are worried about?' before you begin your management plan?

Sometimes, there is a hidden agenda or concern that may be discovered only by allowing the caller this final opportunity to open up, and, if that's the case, this question is exactly what you should ask. It's often your instincts as a clinician that have told you that something just isn't right, despite the lack of red flags being raised during your assessment. This 'gut feeling', which has been developed over time, shouldn't be ignored. We know that many clinical judgements are taken because of the ability we develop as we become experts. When it comes to telephone care, this is more difficult to nurture, as we aren't able to see the patient and recognise when the history doesn't match what we are seeing. Good triagers, however, develop a real gut instinct for when something just doesn't sound right, or the words used don't match what you are hearing, i.e. how the patient sounds. In a way, I am directly contradicting my earlier advice, which was to suggest that you really listen to what is being said. Sometimes, it doesn't matter what you have been told, you just know that the situation, or history, doesn't make total sense. You can't put your finger on it, but something's not right. If you get that kind of reaction (and it could simply be that a mother has said about her child 'I've never seen him like this before'), the safest thing to do is to follow your clinical instinct.

However, the downside to this open question is that you are also allowing the caller to potentially 'hijack' you (see Chapter 6). I have had callers say that their street lights weren't working, or their bins haven't been emptied and could I do anything about it, as well as the usual requests for repeat prescriptions or sick notes.

When you ask such an open question, you are inviting these responses. You may find that you can avoid the potential for having to deal with inappropriate requests by making the question more specific:

Is there anything else about this problem, today, that you think I need to know about?

This helps to keep the conversation confined to the reason for the call, rather than giving permission to ask about anything.

This question also directly links to the initial probing question of 'What were you hoping I'd be able to do for you today?' (see section 4.3, subsection 'Establish the caller's agenda'). If you have established the caller's agenda at the beginning of the call, you shouldn't really need to check again at the end if there is anything else that's worrying them; you should have identified their concerns before you began your assessment.

I understand that this is a difficult point for some clinicians to agree with, but hopefully you will appreciate how this simple question can elongate your call unnecessarily.

Once you have offered your recommendation on what's the best plan of care and it's been agreed (or not, as the case may be – see Chapter 5), you will need to offer 'safety netting' (see section 4.6). But another part of closing the call is providing self-care information. What's the best way to do this?

Self-care advice

Even if you're arranging for a patient to be seen, you may need to offer self-care, also known as 'home care' or 'self-management'. One of the benefits of telephone health care is empowering and educating patients, and this is when we are given the opportunity to either address inappropriate self-care or provide information to enable patients to look after themselves.

One of the criticisms of some commercial triage software programmes is that the clinicians offer too much of the self-care information available to them on their systems and make the call overly long, or they confuse the caller by offering too much information. For some conditions, such as influenza, for instance, there can be pages and pages of self-management information that could be used. This can make the call exceptionally long, both verbally and as far as the call record is concerned. Even though this could be excellent evidence-based information, in the same way that the clinician can be affected by too much information, so can we provide too much self-care information.

One way to make sure you give focused self-care information, while keeping the attention of callers, is to consider saying:

I'm going to give you three key things that you may want to try ...

and then do exactly that. If you feel that they need more than three things, then break it down by saying:

Actually there is a fourth and fifth thing that could help as well. They are ...

By offering things in a numerical order, you help callers with their ability to recall things. It also helps make sure that you stay focused on the principal things to do, rather than bombard callers with lots of less important therapies and lose their attention.

Once you have given the self-care options, you may find it useful to have the caller repeat to you their understanding of what they can try, as we discussed in the chapter on communication. This is especially important if you are recommending or advising any drug treatments.

Once you have discussed self-care management and safety netting (see section 4.6) you need to close the call down quickly and efficiently, without the caller feeling as if you are 'finished with them' and in a hurry to get off the phone.

If you were in the surgery, you would begin to close the consultation by perhaps closing the notes down, handing over the prescription, rising from your chair and walking to the door, giving them their coat and even walking out of the office with the patient to show that you are now going to end the interaction. Over the phone, it's more difficult to indicate that the consultation must now end.

It really just comes down to saying goodbye – easier said than done. Consider developing your own 'script' for saying goodbye such as:

> *Well I hope you are feeling better soon. Thank you for talking to me today. Goodbye.*

Or

> *Thank you for your phone call. I am sure things will get better soon but if not, remember everything we discussed about what to try and when to contact someone if things change or worsen. Goodbye.*

Then you put the phone down. The gold standard within commercial telephone services is that the caller should disconnect first, but, in the clinical world, this can lead to a conversation that goes on and on. As long as you know that you have covered everything and everyone is clear on the next steps (see Chapter 5, section 5.3), you can put the phone down after you have said goodbye.

As we discussed, however, the most important thing to have covered before you disconnect is to check that the caller knows what to do if things change. This is often called 'safety netting', but exactly what does that mean?

4.6 What does safety netting really mean?

How you offer safety netting at the end of the call is probably the most important part of the call and therefore the most important part of this book – especially when you are offering telephone advice only and not seeing your patient. Unfortunately, this is also done very poorly in many calls, as the clinician may not provide enough information on what the continuing risks could be. Good safety netting protects both the patient and the triager.

The weakest form of safety netting is when the triager makes a non-specific offer such as:

Ring back if you are worried about anything at all.

This may seem reasonable, but exactly what does it mean? You are certainly giving callers permission to contact you if they have any concerns, but what should they be concerned about? You're risking receiving calls in which the 'concern' is that they are continuing to experience the same symptoms after a further day, when this was entirely what you would expect, given the disease trajectory – a phone call that is time consuming and unnecessary. Alternatively, and more worryingly, callers or patients may not recognise that something has changed or worsened, and that they need more urgent assistance, and therefore not call anyone. Some patients are reluctant to call for help, despite recognising that something isn't right.

Even if you are arranging a face-to-face consultation [including an emergency response, i.e. a home visit within 1 hour or advising attending A&E (accident and emergency department)], you should consider adding some safety netting regarding what to do if things change or worsen before medical assistance arrives, or before the patient is seen.

So what do we mean when we refer to safety netting? There are three parts to good safety netting that will protect your callers from potential harm and that may also protect you from liability.

These are the three 'W's'.

- *What* they need to look out for (worsening or changing symptoms, including improving). Double-check their understanding of what they have to look out for and don't assume that they have understood everything. Be specific, especially when something has been borderline at the time of the call. When discussing several things, concentrate on the most concerning things, rather than those symptoms that are less critical.
- *When* they should contact someone (the time frame in which to look out for worsening symptoms).
- *Whom* to contact (given the changing symptoms and the time of day).

For instance, say you have just given a parent advice on how to manage a child with symptoms suggesting a non-complex viral infection. Your advice on what to look out for may include increased or excessive vomiting, increased lethargy and worsening temperature, despite antipyretics. This is the 'what to look out for'. You may then advise that the symptoms in their current state may last for up to 3 days, but, if they continue beyond 3 days, or get any worse as discussed during that time (this is the 'when'), they should contact you again. However, if the child's symptoms get worse when the surgery is closed, the parent should call the OOH service (this is the 'whom'). What if the symptoms become more extreme, though, or the parents are worried about meningitis, but there are no red flags at the time of the call? If you have advised that they look out for a petechial rash and neck stiffness ('what to look out for') and these appear, the last thing you want is for them to contact primary care services at any time of day or night. You would advise them to contact 999 services or go to A&E ('whom to contact'), and straight away ('when to contact').

In the case of the elderly, we know that they have very poor uptake of OOH services and so you may want to stress the importance of contacting them (and provide contact details if possible) if the surgery is closed, rather than waiting for the surgery to reopen.

If you have advised self-care and the patient is alone, you may want to consider recommending that someone comes to stay with them. Are they able to call for help if things worsen? Safety netting following telephone advice only, rather than arranging for the patient to be seen, is critical. You need to make sure that callers know exactly what they need to look out for and when to summon help. You may even need to make sure that they have the capacity to do so. I have advised callers to make sure that they keep their phone charged at all times if they are alone, as this is how they would call for help.

I hope that you can see how a simple 'call back if you are worried' doesn't offer much protection. We will discuss the recording of safety netting in your notes in Chapter 7. This is equally important, especially in the absence of voice recordings. However, what should you do if you and the caller can't agree on the outcome?

References

1. Epstein O, Perkin GD, Cookson J, *et al. Clinical Examination.* (4th edn). St Louis, MO: Mosby Elsevier, 2008.
2. Covey SR. *The 7 Habits of Highly Effective People: powerful lessons in personal change.* New York, NY: Simon and Schuster, 1989.
3. Leprohon J, Patel V. Decision-making strategies for telephone triage in emergency medical services. *Medical Decision Making* 1995; **15(3):** 240–53.
4. Wheeler S. *Telephone Triage Protocols for Adult Populations.* (3rd edn). New York, NY: McGraw-Hill Medical, 2009.

Chapter 5

Managing closure

5.1 What if callers won't accept your advice?

Despite your best efforts to offer the safest and most appropriate outcome for your caller and/or patient, there will be times when this advice isn't accepted, or you can't reach a mutually agreeable outcome. So what should you do if this happens?

It's always best to anticipate a potential conflict and have a 'plan B' ready. The second plan, however, must still ensure that patients are as safe as they can be, given their age and the nature of the call. At times, though, we need to accept that we can't be all things to everyone; patients have the right to totally disregard our advice. We have talked about patient demand versus expectation, but sometimes we just can't offer what the patient wants (e.g. a specific appointment time or day). It may be that it's not appropriate, such as a home visit that is unreasonable, given the nature of the complaint and the patient's ability to attend a clinic or surgery. It may be that it's unsafe, such as a request for medication that isn't appropriate. There could be other circumstances, or settings, that make it difficult for patients to comply with your advice, but choosing not to comply is not the same as being unable to comply, as we discussed in the previous chapter.

Let us consider further the situation in which the patient is unable to comply, rather than choosing not to.

There are several conditions in which a patient may be unable to comply with your advice, such as when the patient is:

- a child (reliant on others to accept advice or access health care)
- a young adult (under 18 years of age and able to choose whether to accept your advice or access health care) but with no access to transport or funds for transport

- an elderly person with various issues relating to access to transport, ability to travel and mental capacity
- a person who is socially isolated
- an adult over 18 years of age but lacking transport or funding for transport
- a person who is mentally incapacitated (not elderly)
- a person living in a care facility (and dependent on others to access health care).

Where there are circumstances that make it difficult, or impossible, for patients to manage their own health care, you may find that it is easier to make your decision about what 'plan B' should be based on the age of the patient and/or their mental capacity.

If the patient is a child or someone who cannot make their own decisions, you must stress to the carer the importance of why they need to accept your advice and clearly state the reasons for your advice. Do they understand what may be happening? Have you explained what your differential diagnosis is and the disease trajectory? *You need to clarify whether or not they are making an informed decision.*

For example, say you have just assessed a child that you think has a significant upper respiratory tract infection that needs further examination, but the father is reluctant to bring him into the surgery, as the weather is poor and he has three other children to care for. It's not that he can't get to the surgery, he would just prefer not to. A good way of handling this is to say:

> *From what you have told me, the reason I am suggesting (name the child) is seen within (state the time frame,) is because I can't rule out a chest infection. I would really need to see him to make sure he doesn't require antibiotics or any other treatment. If he doesn't get the right treatment, this could turn into a more significant infection, like pneumonia, and he could become very poorly indeed. I will see (the child) as soon as I can when you arrive; you won't be waiting long.*

The key phrases here are *from what you've told me* – which puts the onus back on to the carer – and *I can't rule out'* – which clearly states what the problem could be (your initial diagnosis). Both of these phrases tell the father that your advice is based on what he has told you, combined with your judgement of what might be occurring, or will occur, if he doesn't bring the child to be seen. Being told that he won't be kept waiting can also act as an incentive. Most carers will respond to this, but, if you are still struggling to gain compliance, remember that your concerns and duty of care are with the child. If a carer still refuses and insists on a home visit, each call should be dealt with on a case-by-case basis. How concerned are you about the child?

If you have advised that a child should be seen within 2 hours, but the carer can't get to the surgery for at least 4 hours owing to transport issues, for instance, what should you do? We discussed the importance of being clear on how long a patient can safely wait to be seen in Chapter 1, section 1.4 (clinical need versus access options), so by now you will be clear on your decision making. If you are certain that a child needs to be seen within 2 hours and that they shouldn't wait any longer than that before being assessed face to face, you have to be very careful about moving the goal posts. If you say 'get here when you can' and hope that it's within the 2 hours you recommended, there is still the risk that it could be up to 4 hours, for example, so how would you stand if the carer turned up 4 hours later with a child that was now severely unwell? In the case of a child, if you have made a clinical judgement that they need further care and assessment within a certain time frame and the child can't get to you, *you may need to go to the child.* In a busy practice, this may not always seem reasonable. You have other patients and other duties to take care of. Perhaps there is a walk-in centre or an urgent care centre nearer to the child that the parent can get to more easily? Failing that, depending on the severity of the illness, you may even want to consider arranging transport to hospital, but this is extreme and wouldn't be necessary if primary care is what is needed. If the parent doesn't choose to comply with your advice, your plan B will depend on your reasons for wanting to see the child and how quickly. Many clinicians will say that, as long as they are clear about worsening symptoms, it's then the carers' responsibility to bring children in when they can. I understand this, but, if you felt that a child needed to be seen within 2 hours, why? It would be very difficult to say, 'It wasn't my fault' if something awful happened, as you assessed the need for the child to be seen within 2 hours, but then didn't make sure that that happened. Would your duty of care be called into question?

I have known some services to say that when carers refuse to bring children to be seen and insist on a home visit (an inappropriate level of care), they could arguably be reported to social services. Denying children access to health care, i.e. they are able to bring the child to the surgery and travelling will not cause the child to deteriorate but they choose not to do so, could be interpreted in this way. Having said that this option was available to clinical staff, it was very rarely put into practice, as it was easier to capitulate than report carers to social services. One service, however, had significant success with this strategy and reduced the number of home visits. Clinicians will always want to make sure that children receive the care they need first and foremost. In addition, the threat of involving social services could cause irreparable damage to the relationship with the carer and even result in a lack of future contact, which could be a risk for the child. I also understand why these measures could become necessary, as some carers can completely misuse the home visiting service. Inappropriate home visits can put other patients and clinicians at risk: patients may wait even longer for a home visit than necessary and clinical staff are put at risk when carrying out home visits in bad weather or busy traffic.

This is, of course, an extreme way of handling inappropriate requests for home visits, but, if you are worried about a child, you may need to use these tactics to gain cooperation. There is no easy way to resolve the issue of when and where children should be seen and, as we have discussed, you will need to make an individual decision each time, based on your knowledge of the child, the carer and the social circumstances, as well as the resources available to you. The overriding factor should always be 'what's best for the child'. As much as a carer may be misusing the service, if you are worried about the wellbeing of a child, your decision should always be to ensure his or her safety first. You may wish to seek further advice on the handling of this situation from local leads, the organisation in which you work or even your indemnity provider. Safeguarding children is our primary concern and you should always ensure that they receive the care needed, either by clearly stipulating what the consequences could be of a failure to follow advice or by seeing children at home, even when this may not be clinically appropriate.

When it comes to adults, however, your tactics will be different. If you are sure that they need a face-to-face assessment and are clear about the time frame, if patients can't get to you, or travelling may cause them to deteriorate and you are concerned about that, you may have to go to them. But what about when the patient is a competent adult and travelling will not cause them to decline? Does the same duty of care apply?

We will discuss whether you have done enough in the next section, but another way to gain patients' cooperation (especially when they won't accept a higher level of care) is what nurses often refer to as a 'duty to terrify'! Personally, I have used this kind of approach several times with elderly patients who have refused an ambulance when they have described symptoms suggesting a cardiac event:

From what you've told me, I can't rule out the possibility of a heart attack. If you don't let me arrange an ambulance straight away, you may die.

If they still decline, I will then say:

As I said, from what you told me was happening, you could be having a heart attack. Are you sure I can't arrange an ambulance for you?

At this point they usually agree, but if they don't, and there is no reason to suspect any mental capacity issues, I will finish by saying:

'OK, I will make a note of the fact that I have strongly advised an ambulance as I suspect a possible heart attack and you have declined it.

Make it clear to callers or patients that you are documenting their decision not to acquiesce ('declining' is a less confrontational way of saying it than 'refused'), but it is their right to do so. At this point, however, you may find that they'll accept your advice.

In summary, this is a very difficult situation to manage, so by always thinking of the patient's safety first, you may find your decision making easier. If you are worried about a patient and they won't come to you, you will need to consider what could happen if they don't get care within your recommended time frame – but, is there anything else you can do?

5.2 Have you done enough?

If you advise an adult to be seen but he or she refuses to accept your outcome, should you then capitulate with a home visit when it isn't appropriate?

If patients are capable of accessing the care you have recommended but refuse to do so, as long as they understand why you have reached your conclusion and understand the consequences of not accessing the care advised, then the choice is theirs. The key here, is to *ensure that they are making an informed decision.* This is particularly important if they refuse a face-to-face consultation and prefer to self-manage, or see someone within a time frame that is outside your recommendation.

For example, say you have assessed an adult with symptoms of a significant chest infection and you recommend that they be seen that day, but they tell you they feel too unwell to attend, or they prefer to come down the next day or be seen by their own GP at a later time, what would you do?

You should explain that you can't rule out a chest infection that may require treatment, otherwise it could become very serious and even develop into pneumonia if left untreated. If the patient still refuses to take your advice, then that is his or her decision. If you don't explain the reasons and the consequences, however, you aren't allowing the patient to make an informed decision, which may make you liable for the outcome.

There have been cases in which patients have been offered a face-to-face consultation in the surgery or clinic but have declined (typically it happens with OOH care) and, when they become very unwell (unfortunately even dying), the family has accused the clinicians of neglect, as they didn't arrange a home visit. In my opinion, if a patient declines to come to see a clinician when they are capable of doing so (to clarify, this means that they are physically capable of attending the surgery and doing so would not result in further deterioration of their condition) and it has been clearly explained to them why they need to be seen and what may happen if they don't accept the clinician's advice, it is then the patient's responsibility if they choose to ignore that advice. Where the clinician has any doubt about the patient's capacity to make an informed decision, however, or there is the potential for the patient's condition to deteriorate by travelling, it could be argued that the clinician has a duty of care to go to the patient, i.e. carry out a home visit or, if that isn't possible within the appropriate time frame owing to other service requirements, perhaps arranging transport to hospital may be necessary.

In the case of a child, as discussed in the previous section, the clinician has a duty to the child. If the parents or carers decline to bring a child to be seen within the time frame clinically relevant to the child's condition at the time of the call, the clinician must think first and foremost of the child. If he or she needs to be seen, plan B may be to make a home visit or recommend another care facility closer to home.

The key message here is *don't change your outcome (e.g. see within 2 hours changes to see 'whenever possible'), when the patient's ability to get to you is the issue.* If the parent or carer chooses not to transport the patient within the time frame you recommended and that was agreed, I would suggest that you can't be held responsible.

Another important issue, after you have agreed the outcome with the caller, is to establish what is going to happen next. Have you clearly ascertained that?

5.3 Is everyone clear about what happens next?

Once you and callers or patients appear to have reached an outcome and you have been very clear on what that means to them, i.e. informed decision making, it's essential that you and callers are clear on what the next steps are to be. I have had many callers who have accepted 'self-care' and, after spending a couple of minutes talking through what they should do to manage the symptoms, they have then asked, 'That's great and when do I see the doctor?' Obviously I wasn't as clear as I thought I had been in explaining what was going to happen!

However, when the outcome has been clearly explained and accepted, what about any follow-up arrangements? Does the caller understand what will happen next? In many cases, you may want to review the patient at a later time, but you feel that this can be done with a follow-up phone call. Have you explained this clearly and has it been understood by the caller that you want to know how things are, but it will be a second phone call and not a face-to-face appointment? Conversely, what if you want to see the patient to follow up, but the patient thinks that you will phone to find out how they are doing?

Once you have decided on what the next steps should be, make sure that you explain them clearly to patients and that they have interpreted your advice correctly. You may want to say something along these lines:

> *Just to make sure we both understand what's going to happen next/when I will speak to you again, would you mind telling me what I said? I want to make sure I was clear in the way I explained it.*

Remember the section on communication and getting callers to repeat to you their understanding? The same technique is useful here.

Once you and callers are clear on the next steps, it's equally important that you record the details in their notes. Unless you are pre-booking a review yourself, there is often one other person involved in the next steps – the receptionist. Many patients, despite your clarification that the next review will be over the phone, will forget that and contact the surgery to arrange a face-to-face appointment. They will tell the receptionist, 'The doctor wanted to see me again in a week's time, so I need an appointment for then.'

Where you are operating a 'total triage system' (see Chapter 10), it's vitally important that everyone is clear on the next steps by documenting clearly what has been agreed. When the patient then phones and asks for a face-to-face appointment in a week's time, the receptionists can look at the notes and see what was agreed. If a telephone review was the outcome, they will then know to book a telephone call, rather than an appointment, by saying:

> *Oh yes, I can see when you spoke to/saw the GP last time, she's written in your notes that she would like to speak to you again in a week's time. Could you ring back on (date) and arrange a call-back for that day? Don't worry, if you need to be seen, the GP will arrange that for you that day.*

If you aren't operating a total triage system, the receptionist could say:

> *I can see in your notes the GP has said she would like to review you over the phone next time. I'm going to book a call-back for you on (date). If you need to be seen that day after the phone call, don't worry. The GP can arrange that for you.*

It is always a much more efficient system to empower your receptionists to look at patients' notes to see what the agreed next steps were, otherwise many patients will take a face-to-face appointment when a quick phone call might have sufficed. This is just one of the pitfalls that can be encountered when communicating the next steps. What other pitfalls might you encounter?

Chapter 6

Common pitfalls

6.1 What are the pitfalls?

Throughout the previous chapters we have discussed many of the pitfalls you might encounter when it comes to telephone assessments. There are so many pitfalls that this could be a book in itself, but let's look at some of the most common ones you might come across.

Triaging without the patient present

This is so easily done, especially when the call is placed by a third party and particularly in the case of a child. Remember to ask the three key questions (section 4.3):

- Where is the patient?
- What are they doing?
- How does the patient seem to the third party?

There is then less risk of your finding out too late that the patient isn't present. Triaging without the patient can lead to mistriage and can be very dangerous. In some instances, you may still need to progress with your assessment even without the patient, as some advice may be safer than no advice. For example, when I first started doing telephone triage, many households did not have a phone and parents would come out to a phone box in the middle of the night seeking advice about their child, who was at home. This would rarely happen nowadays with the advent of mobile phones, but it is still possible. How accurate can the assessment be if they aren't with the child at the time of the call? If you feel that you need to attempt an assessment, you may want to say:

As you aren't with (name the child) I can only offer an assessment based on the information you can provide. Please understand this may not be sufficient and, in that case, we will talk about the safest plan of action. I will do my best to help, but if you aren't able to tell me what's happening at this exact moment in time, we may need to do something, such as you bringing (name the child) in. Let's see what we can do though first.

However, in some cases I would refuse to carry out an assessment in the absence of the patient, as it wouldn't be safe to offer advice on what could be totally inaccurate information. I would then say:

I am very sorry but it wouldn't be safe for me to give you advice when you aren't with the patient, as the information you give me might not be accurate. The safest thing to do would be to either call back when you are with the patient, or take them to a care facility, such as A&E or a walk-in centre, for further advice.

Don't be bullied into giving advice when it can't be done safely. Go with the safest option, or arrange a call-back when the patient can be present. This might include calling the person who is with the patient, rather than the person who placed the call, e.g. if the child is with one parent but another called you for advice. Can you ring the parent who is currently with the child? In addition, be very wary of offering advice when the patient is unaware of the call. Many adults will phone a GP about their concerns regarding their elderly parents. If they aren't with them at the time of the call, be careful of offering advice based on potentially outdated information, or of course about anything that could be considered confidential.

'Hijacking'
This is the term that describes when you are just about to end the call and the caller says 'While I have you ...' or 'Could I also just ask you about ...' and you end up discussing something else and lose control of the call. It could also be because you have asked, 'Is there anything else I can help you with or you're worried about?'

If you clarify the reason for calls at the beginning and ask callers what they hope you will be able to do for them, as discussed in section 4.3, you shouldn't get 'hijacked' too often. If you suspect that a caller is likely to do this, make sure that you clarify with them again at the beginning of the call what they wish to talk to you about and perhaps say:

So, just to be clear, we are going to talk about ... Are you sure there wasn't anything else you wanted to talk about today?

If callers still surprise you at the end of the call, you can decide if it's appropriate to continue to talk about another issue, or remind them that you asked them what they needed to discuss at the beginning and they failed to mention a second issue then. You can then suggest that they can either place another call, or discuss the second issue when you see them, if they are coming to see you.

To a certain extent, being hijacked can be your own fault. If you have made it clear at the beginning what the call will involve, but then choose to allow the caller to take control, by talking about other issues, you may have to live with the consequences.

Triaging 'irrelevant' information

We have looked at clarifying the chief complaint and the reason for the call, but it's still possible to triage what is, essentially, irrelevant information. The caller may briefly mention something that you then feel duty bound to probe further. This is why it's so important that you spend time establishing the reason for the call and differentiating between the chief complaint and associated symptoms. We talked about when to probe and when to pursue in Chapter 3, but, when it comes to triaging extraneous information, we need to be mindful of giving time to discussing what's been happening, without going into detail about something that, at the time of the call, is unimportant. The question you will be asking now, though, is 'How do we know if it's important or not?', as the danger is, of course, that you may hear something that you feel is irrelevant and it turns out to be of real importance.

The skill in telephone triage is not to rush too quickly into the assessment before finding out what's really going on. Also, we need to be careful about the way we ask questions, as we can lead the caller into giving us information that isn't relevant. If you ask a caller about a headache and their response indicates that they realise that they did have one *only after* being prompted, this doesn't mean to say the headache wasn't there, but how much of an issue was it at the time if the caller didn't volunteer the information?

If you suspect that callers may not even realise the relevance of some symptoms, try spending more time probing into what's been happening, how they are managing to function and any other symptoms that they've noticed (all open questions) rather than a straightforward 'Do you have ...' (closed question).

Just because callers haven't mentioned something specifically doesn't mean that it isn't happening, as we know, but, if you have given them several opportunities to mention something, but they still don't and it then turns out to be important, the key question that will be asked of you is 'Did you make every effort to find out?'. The poorest response that you can give is, 'They didn't tell me about it', unless you have allowed them the opportunity to mention something, or asked enough questions to try to find out if it was an issue for them.

For example, let's say that you are talking to a patient who has abdominal pain and you ask if they have any medical history. They give you a negative response, but it turns out that they have adhesions caused by abdominal surgery. If this was a potential cause of abdominal pain, you should have asked specifically if they'd had any surgery at any time. Many patients don't see routine surgery as 'medical history'. Some patients with an ongoing health complaint will still answer 'No' when asked if they have any medical problems. If it's something that could be a factor in explaining symptoms, or ruling out a diagnosis, you should ask specifically about it (without leading, if possible), even if they insist that they don't have any problems. If we don't have access to someone's medical history, we can sometimes be a better triager – if it's relevant, we should ask about it, rather than relying on callers to offer the information.

Even if callers have a complex history, or long-term medical conditions, such as diabetes, it's too easy to look at their history and get taken off track by what's happened in the past. If it's relevant at the time of the call, ask about it. If it's not relevant, leave it for another time.

Not checking medication

One of the common pitfalls when triaging patients is a failure to clarify what medications have been taken, or how much. We can rely too much on patients' records but, when we have no access to that information, we can also make assumptions about medications. For instance, when parents say that they have given their child a 'teaspoon' of medicine, we may assume that it is 5 mL, but, if we fail to check what a 'teaspoon' is, patients can receive too little a dose or, more worryingly, be overdosed. Adults will say that they have taken 'some paracetamol', which can mean anything from one to ten tablets. We have a duty to ensure that we know exactly what has been tried and how often. In addition, don't forget about over-the-counter medications that could be contraindicated. In the elderly, many complaints are related to interactions between medicines; they may try a friend's medicine, as it worked for the friend, or they may buy something from a health food shop that is contraindicated. As a triager, you should ensure that you know exactly what has been tried (see Chapter 4, section 4.3) and also what you can then safely offer by way of medication.

Over-investing in the caller's assessment or trivialising their concerns

There is the potential for either overplaying or exaggerating, or, conversely, underplaying of symptoms to confirm or exclude a diagnosis on the telephone.[1] The elderly can underplay their symptoms by 'not wanting to bother the doctor'. Others may exaggerate their symptoms in order to gain access to a health provider when it is not necessary.

The 'wrong train syndrome'[2]

This means that, no matter how fast you travel, if you go to the wrong platform, you'll never get to the right place! In other words, don't jump to conclusions too quickly or steam ahead without constantly making sure that you are on the same page as your caller. *Never assume anything* – check out all details and responses.

Leading questions

Leading questions are often associated with time constraints. By suggesting to callers what you want their responses to be, your consultation will be quicker, but you may arrive at completely the wrong conclusion and miss something vital. Poor triages often contain several leading questions. If you are able to listen to voice recordings of calls, see if there is any correlation between the length of the call and the types of questions asked. Do shorter calls have more leading or more closed questions?

These are just some of the most common pitfalls you are in danger of encountering. Another common pitfall is in relation to documentation or record keeping – it can be overly long, far too brief or inaccurate. So what's best practice when it comes to record keeping?

References

1. Foster J, Jessop L, Dale J. Concerns and confidence of general practitioners in providing telephone consultations. *British Journal of General Practice* 1999; **49**: 111–13.
2. Clawson JJ, Dernocoeur KB. *Principles of Emergency Medical Dispatch: how EMD should be practiced in modern public safety.* (3rd edn). Salt Lake City, UT: National Academies of EMD, 2004.

Chapter 7

Record keeping

7.1 How much should you document?

When it comes to telephone triage, you may have two or three forms of documentation: an electronic document, a hand-written record and possibly a voice recording of the call.

As with all types of care, record keeping must be of the highest standard and must comply with legislation. In the UK the relevant legislation includes the Data Protection Act,[1] the Freedom of Information Act,[2] the General Medical Council's (GMC's) guidance on good medical practice[3] and the Nursing and Midwifery Council's (NMC's) *Code for Nurses and Midwives*.[4] The NMC Code 2015 states:

> *10. Keep clear and accurate records relevant to your practice.*
> *This includes but is not limited to patient records. It includes all records that are relevant to your scope of practice.*

In 1998 the GMC stated that 'providing advice and medical services by telephone shouldn't diminish the quality of the care patients receive'. This was later withdrawn with the advent of remote prescribing guidelines, but it is probably still a best practice guide.

The GMC's *Good Medical Practice* (2013) guidance[3] states:

> *Record your work clearly, accurately and legibly.*
> *19. Documents you make (including clinical records) to formally record your work must be clear, accurate and legible.*
> *You should make records at the same time as the events you are recording or as soon as possible afterwards.*

20. You must keep records that contain personal information about patients, colleagues or others securely, and in line with any data protection requirements.
21. Clinical records should include:
(a) relevant clinical findings
(b) the decisions made and actions agreed, and who is making the decisions and agreeing the actions
(c) the information given to patients
(d) any drugs prescribed or other investigation or treatment
(e) who is making the record and when.

Both the guidelines and the Code are designed primarily with written and/ or electronic records in mind, but voice recordings of telephone conversations are now an accepted form of record keeping as far as the NMC and the GMC are concerned. However, voice recordings can still get lost, become corrupt or be of poor quality and so should never be relied on solely. The electronic or hand-written record must provide enough information to support your telephone consultation and outcome and should be written in such a way that it will provide enough evidence, without having to rely on the voice recording as backup.

In the interests of clarity, 'documentation' from this point forward will refer to the electronic or hand-written record unless indicated otherwise.

Your documentation is one of the key components protecting you from legal liability. In the absence of visually or physically confirming the history you have taken and the clinical findings, your documentation needs to be sufficient to support your actions and to potentially defend you if things go wrong. At the same time, you need to balance the amount of documentation with the time you have available. You have to be efficient in your documentation, without feeling the need to write out everything that was discussed or mentioned.

Do the same documentation principles apply to a telephone triage as they would to a face-to-face encounter? Well let's think about that. Do you write out the full conversation that you have when seeing a patient? I would suggest that you don't – you'll document the salient points, the clinical findings and your actions/treatment/outcome. So perhaps the same approach should apply to a phone call? The one element that is missing is your physical examination, but the majority of the consultation is exactly the same – history taking. We have discussed how this is exactly the same in both a face-to-face encounter and a phone consultation, so the same documentation standards will apply. However, in the absence of physical or visual confirmation of our differential diagnosis, we need to document information that would replace them. An example would be what you asked the caller to do with regard to taking a temperature, or making other checks, e.g. response to pressing on an area of abdominal pain, positioning issues or putting the chin to the chest. Any findings from this type of questioning may need to be documented *if they are relevant.*

The best thing to do regarding your documentation is to have a system or protocol, in the same way as you do for your call structure, but one that can be flexible depending on the nature of the call. If you are using a clinical decision support system (CDSS), your documentation will be structured according to the system you are using, but there will always be an option to enter free text. This is often when documentation is either missed or repeated, given that the information has been recorded elsewhere. Where there aren't restrictions or templates to work within, you must ensure that your documentation is succinct without being too brief, detailed but relevant and, of course, an accurate reflection of the conversation. Unfortunately, I have listened to calls with the accompanying call record or documentation in front of me and I have asked myself if I have the right record, as it doesn't reflect the call I am listening to. Alternatively, some documentation can be so brief, such as 'Appointment given' or 'To be seen', that I have no idea at all what happened during the call. What if the patient didn't turn up for the appointment and there wasn't any form of voice recording? In that case, clinicians would be completely vulnerable when it comes to defending themselves if something untoward happened to the patient. Some clinicians would maintain that there is little point in writing out a full history when they're seeing the patient, but I would still argue that this type of 'efficiency' is dangerous. How would you defend yourself if something went wrong?

Documentation can also vary according to who triages and who then sees the patient. When doing both the triage and the face-to-face consultation, there is the temptation to think, 'I'll write everything up when I see them.' Alternatively, when not seeing patients themselves, clinicians may think that they need to write absolutely everything out in full to justify why they have arranged a further consultation. So what's the right balance? Is there a minimum amount that you should document?

7.2 What are the minimum criteria for record keeping?

As discussed in the previous section, getting the balance right between too little and too much documentation is tricky. We need to make sure that everyone is clear about why we acted in the way we did, without taking so much time to document the call that we are adding to our workload unnecessarily and losing some of the efficiencies that we know are a benefit of telephone health care.

When it comes to record keeping, there are some criteria or documentation standards that you may want to consider to help maximise efficiency, without risking incomplete or inaccurate documentation. As with the triage model, these criteria can be adapted to the nature of the call and every criterion may not be required in all calls.

Documentation criteria

Make it clear that the call was a telephone interaction

It's surprising how often an interaction on the patient record appears to be a face-to-face consultation, when it was actually a phone consultation. If your system is designed to default to one or the other automatically, you need to make sure that the interaction has been accurately recorded as a phone consultation.

Whom you spoke to

If you spoke to anyone other than the patient and were given any information at all on the condition of the patient, or the history of the reason for the contact, make sure that you document whom you spoke to and what information they gave you. If possible, obtain their name but, failing that, their relationship to the caller. If you have observed all of the confidentiality issues, you should know whom you are talking to anyway.

An overview or synopsis of the call

It doesn't have to be long and complicated, but make sure that you have documented what the call was about. What was the chief complaint? Document the duration and location of the problem and any treatments tried and their effect, where appropriate. Think about the history you have taken and what information from the 'symptom and patient' history would support your outcome – that is what should be documented.

This is another system that may be useful:

- when advising self-care management and not arranging for someone to be seen, document what was answered in the negative, e.g. 'Not seeing them because symptoms/signs A, B and C weren't present'

- when arranging a face-to-face consultation, document what was answered in the positive, e.g. 'Getting them seen because symptoms/signs X, Y and Z were present'.

This may help to focus your documentation rather than writing out 'They had ... symptoms/signs A, B and C but didn't have symptoms/signs X, Y and Z.' In addition, if you are questioned about why something may not have been written down, by being able to explain your documentation system you can defend why it wasn't documented. For example, say a patient has had symptoms of flu that included reference to a headache, but at the time of the call that wasn't a suspicious symptom or a red flag. Later on he or she develops a much more severe headache, suggesting a septic infection. If asked why you hadn't documented the presence of a headache, even though it was discussed, you would be able to respond that your call record-keeping system, when not referring a patient to a face-to-face consultation, would document only what had been answered in the negative, or had no clinical importance at the time of the call. If it wasn't documented, it wasn't relevant to your clinical judgement and decision making and therefore to the outcome.

Alternatively, if you were having a patient referred on for a face-to-face consultation but you were later questioned about why you hadn't documented whether a symptom had been present at the time of the call, you would be able to state that your documentation system would, when referring onwards, include only symptoms that had been present during the call. Therefore, if it had not been documented, it must not have been present.

In summary, if having a patient seen, focus on what was answered in the positive. If the patient is not going to be seen, focus on what was answered in the negative. There may be exceptions to this, but this simple rule could help to reduce your documentation. The key message here is to be able to state very clearly what your documentation process is, so that you can defend why something was or, more importantly, wasn't included.

Past medical history (PMH), medications (including over-the-counter medications) and allergies

These are questions that should always be asked (see Chapter 4, section 4.3) and documented as having been asked, along with the response given. They are vital when it comes to supporting your level of advice in the absence of a voice recording. If prescribing or advising medication, ensure that you document what allergies were present and, if necessary, any warnings you may have given about contraindications or reactions.

Self-care information

All self-care information and medication advice should be documented in full. This would include dosage of any medications advised, e.g. '1 g of paracetamol to be taken immediately, but no more than 4 g in 24 hours'. If you have decided not to follow NICE (National Institute for Health and Care Excellence) guidelines, you may need to document why. If you have been able to refer the caller to a website for additional self-care information, document which one.

Specific safety-netting advice

Full safety-netting advice should be documented in case the caller denies the instructions given for contacting you again, or chooses not to follow your advice about going to A&E (the accident and emergency department), for instance. We discussed safety netting in detail in Chapter 4, section 4.6, and its documentation needs to be equally robust. In the same way that safety netting can be done in a very non-specific way ('Call back if you're worried'), so too can its documentation. Don't skip over this crucial part of your documentation. Provide details on what you advised, or where you referred the caller for additional information. If something goes wrong following a triage, and the call isn't recorded, this will be one of the biggest points of contention. Did you fully protect your patient with clear safety-netting instructions? See section 7.4 for further information on documenting safety netting. Providing good safety netting protects the patient, but the documentation of the safety netting protects the triager.

What the caller plans to do

Whether or not the caller has agreed with your recommended advice, document exactly what he or she plans to do. Occasionally, callers may not agree to attend a face-to-face consultation and may even deny what was advised. If callers disagree with you at all, document what they said they were going to do. In addition, for the purposes of ensuring that anyone else involved in the patient's care understands your decision making, it's important that you have documented your advice and the caller's choice. For instance, if you have tried to offer self-care management but the caller insists on seeing someone, document clearly what you advised and why, so that any other clinicians involved will understand why the patient has received an appointment when it may not have been clinically appropriate. If it turns out that the patient should have been seen and you had missed something, you could receive feedback that will help in future consultations.

Any referral or follow-up arrangements

Ensure that you document what follow-up arrangements have been made. Include place of referral, names of anyone you have directly referred the patient to and the time the referral was made or the time of the face-to-face consultation. Document whether callers were advised to attend A&E within 1 hour or, if advised to see their GP, what time frame was suggested, i.e. was an urgent appointment advised or the next available routine appointment (depending on the appointment system)? If arranging an ambulance, try to get the reference number.

I know of two cases in which hospital staff denied any knowledge of accepting patients for admission from an out-of-hours (OOH) service. This was compounded by the fact that there was no record in the patients' notes of who the receiving doctors had been. However, the calls had been voice recorded and we were able to provide evidence that proper procedures had been followed. This was an unnecessary waste of time that could have been avoided if the GP referring the patient had taken a name and documented the time of the call.

This is just one example of where the voice recording has been used, but is recording calls really worth it?

7.3 Should you voice record your calls?

Recording of calls is becoming more prevalent in telephone triage and certainly more so in OOH service providers, which will typically record all interactions for quality control and training purposes. But it's still uncommon in general practice and most other telephone services. So what are the real advantages?

There are several reasons why I would recommend recording calls:

1 for continuous professional development (CPD) purposes
2 for training purposes
3 for use in clinical audit or quality assurance, including clinical governance
4 as a non-invasive way of recording interactions that helps both patients and clinicians
5 to potentially moderate the behaviour of callers and/or clinicians
6 to save time and money when it comes to investigating complaints.

It must be noted at this point that call recordings can be made only with the permission of the caller. This is a legal requirement (see section 7.4).

Let's look in more detail at the advantages of voice recording.

CPD purposes

There is nothing more powerful than listening to your own calls to help you with your own learning and development. You can hear very easily what you do well and what might need tweaking or improving. For instance, you may realise that you have a habit of talking over the top of callers, or that you're silent too much without explaining your actions. You will hear how your tone is really coming across and how it may be affecting the interaction. It can help with your call management, as you might find that you are struggling to say goodbye, or you need to tighten up on your introduction. Most importantly, it can help improve your call structure, which is one of the biggest problems within telephone triage.

If you have access to voice recordings made by fellow clinicians, it's always a worthwhile exercise to listen to each other's calls and provide feedback. This could be clinical supervision for nurses or peer review. Listening to calls taken by others can greatly enhance your practice. You may have been struggling for years with how to approach a question, and then you may hear someone else address it in a way you hadn't thought of.

Training purposes

From an organisational point of view, access to call recordings will greatly improve your ability to train staff and to monitor their progress. Giving feedback retrospectively via voice recordings, is often more effective than 'live' feedback. Sitting alongside someone taking a call can affect their behaviour and performance, making them very self-conscious and therefore less natural in their approach. You also have the opportunity to replay calls if you have any doubt about what was discussed, whereas, with live monitoring, you could have misheard something or misinterpreted something and then given inaccurate feedback.

If clinicians are being observed for poor performance, voice recordings are invaluable as a method of monitoring their practice. Once again, you can use listening to calls as a method for training, i.e. you could ask a clinician to listen to other people's calls as part of a performance management plan, or have examples of calls that demonstrate certain learning points.

I have found access to voice recordings the singular most important tool when it comes to training staff. It demonstrates clearly many of the important issues such as tone of voice, sending/receiving information, communication issues, call structure and managing calls effectively. None of this is apparent from the documentation of the call alone.

Clinical audit and quality assurance

If you are giving or receiving more formal feedback, call recordings make this far more attainable. When it comes to the quality assurance of calls in general practice there aren't any requirements for in hours, but there are standards for OOH services (see Chapter 8). Access to voice recordings makes any audit more accurate and accessible. When presenting feedback, the evidence on the voice recording may be irrefutable, but there is also a level of subjectivity when it comes to tone of voice, for instance.

Audit via voice recordings also allows the auditor to do the work remotely, rather than being on site, which can make for more cost-effective practice.

Finally, if you are in the unfortunate position of being criticised for the outcome or your handling of a call and there is a discrepancy in your documentation, or a situation in which the caller denies that you told them something, you can ultimately defend yourself with a voice recording. I have found that the voice recordings usually defend the clinician rather than condemn them, but that is always a possibility.

You might like to consider using an audit tool specifically designed for auditing clinicians' telephone interactions, as it is much more appropriate to use a tool than non-specific feedback. We will discuss clinical audit and quality assurance in more depth in Chapter 8, as it is an essential part of telephone services.

A non-invasive way of recording an interaction

There are very few areas in medicine where we are able to record the interaction between a clinician and a patient in such a non-invasive way. Video recording can often be uncomfortable for either party and it can affect the interaction. The recording of a phone call can help the clinician in the ways outlined above and if there are discrepancies between the patient and the clinician, playing the call for the patient can resolve some of these issues very quickly.

Moderating the behaviours of callers and/or clinicians

It is lamentable, I know, but when either the caller or the clinician is reminded that the call is being recorded, it can moderate behaviour. I have heard callers verbally abusing clinicians, but, when they are reminded of the fact the call is being recorded, they not only stop the abuse but also apologise for their behaviour. Unfortunately, I also know of a case in which a caller, who was notorious for verbally abusing staff, made a complaint that a clinician had sworn at him. The surgery immediately defended the clinician, but said that it would listen to the call. The clinician in question had forgotten that calls were voice recorded and when pushed to the limit by a very unpleasant patient, had finally snapped. He was heard to use inappropriate language to the abusive patient (probably for the first time in his career). I know that this behaviour was iniquitous, but we have all been tempted at times to say things that aren't appropriate when dealing with abusers of the system and staff. Knowing that we are being recorded can sometimes help to keep our own behaviour moderated, even when being pushed to the extreme.

It saves time and money when it comes to investigating complaints

If there is a complaint or an untoward incident as a result of a telephone interaction, having access to the voice recording can save hours, if not days or even weeks, in terms of the time required to answer the complaint. This, in turn, can save thousands of pounds.

If you are currently considering recording calls, but are hesitating because you may have to change phone systems, which can incur significant expense, I would urge you to consider the costs that may be required when something goes wrong or when there is a complaint. When you hear the voice recording, you can often make an immediate decision on whether or not the clinician acted appropriately, rather than asking for statements, reviewing the notes, responding to the complainant, getting other services involved if it's not resolved locally, and so on. I can't recommend voice recording calls highly enough, but what do you need to consider from a legal point of view when it comes to all forms of record keeping?

7.4 Where do you stand medicolegally?

When it comes to voice recordings, as we know, they are admissible in court, but your primary care record, for the purposes of record keeping, is your electronic record. In the absence of a voice recording, where do you stand medicolegally as far as your documentation is concerned?

A frequently asked question is – 'Is it true that, "if it's not written down, it did not happen"?'. This isn't literally true, of course; simply because it hasn't been recorded doesn't mean it wasn't discussed or done. However, from a legal standpoint this may very well be regarded as factual. If it hasn't been documented and you aren't able to prove what was discussed from a voice recording, your governing body or a court may decide that you could be liable.

When it comes to the accuracy of your records, if there is a discrepancy between your notes and what the caller recalls, whom will your governing body side with?

The NMC says the following:

> Courts of law tend to adopt the approach that 'if it is not recorded, it has not been done'.

and

> You must use your professional judgement to decide what is relevant and should be recorded.

The GMC will take a similar stance, namely that, in the absence of being able to demonstrate what you discussed in your documentation, it may very well accept the caller's version of events.

It is advisable to document anything that you require to support your decision making if voice recordings are unavailable (see section 7.2). In particular, remember to consider your documentation of the safety-netting advice given (see Chapter 4, section 4.6).

Telephone triage is now an accepted form of remote assessment. The medicolegal aspects of this work are the same as any other form of medical or nursing practice, but there is a lack of specific guidance when it comes to telephone triage. The usual best practice regarding accessing training, keeping yourself up to date and knowing when you have exceeded your professional boundaries remain. However, I think that one of the most worrying aspects of this work is that many practitioners don't recognise that there are specific skills required, and that being a qualified doctor or nurse doesn't mean that you have the ability, or knowledge, to carry out telephone consultations. Wherever you are working, I would ask that you question your ability to work in this difficult and immensely risky area. If you haven't undertaken any training, please do so. Even if you have been doing telephone triage for years, I would urge you to attend some training. However, please research who is offering the training to ensure that it is of good quality, as, like the skill itself, training can come in many forms. I have personal experience of attending someone else's training event (with a view to my own CPD), and it was one of the least useful things I have ever done. It would be unprofessional of me to name the organisation that provided it. Almost everyone I have ever had the opportunity to teach, even though they may have been doing telephone triage for years, if not decades, has agreed that they thought they knew what they were doing, but they realised after our training session that there was so much more to telephone triage.

One of the best ways to ensure that you are following best practice is to review your calls, both voice recordings and documentation and to ensure that they are quality assured. However, should you go as far as 'auditing' your calls, and what does that mean?

References

1. UK Parliament. Data Protection Act 1998. London: TSO, www.legislation.gov.uk/ukpga/1998/29/contents [accessed 28 September 2016].
2. UK Parliament. Freedom of Information Act 2000. London: TSO, www.legislation.gov.uk/ukpga/2000/36/contents [accessed 28 September 2016].
3. General Medical Council. *Good Medical Practice*. London: GMC, 2013, www.gmc-uk.org/guidance/good_medical_practice.asp [accessed 28 September 2016].
4. Nursing and Midwifery Council. *The Code for Nurses and Midwives*. London: NMC, www.nmc.org.uk/standards/ [accessed 28 September 2016].

Chapter 8

Clinical audit

8.1 Should you audit your calls?

It has been suggested[1] that quality assurance and audit checks should be made to help protect nurses against legal liability when carrying out telephone triage. This could equally apply to doctors, but it is not typically part of everyday general practice.

So, why should we consider auditing/reviewing our calls? Some of the main benefits and advantages are:

- it improves patient care and safety
- it provides feedback and learning for clinicians and therefore improves skills and confidence
- it informs employers who is best at telephone triage or which practitioners are giving rise to cause for concern
- it can help make a service more cost-effective and improve performance through good-quality consultations as a result of regular feedback
- it can identify where resources are needed.

Some of the disadvantages are:

- it can be time consuming
- it can be expensive to carry out, as significant resources are needed
- it can be poorly received (if not done well or efficiently)
- it can result in expensive changes being required
- it can identify unsafe practice, which then requires further action (which is also time consuming and expensive).

In the UK there isn't any legislation that requires quality monitoring of telephone consultations [except within out-of-hours (OOH) services], and it is not standard practice in most organisations. It is neither expected, nor preferred, as part of quality assuring telephone services. This is understandable to a certain extent, but we are now looking at the quality of the care delivered in general practice. At the time of writing, practices in the UK use the Quality and Outcomes Framework (QOF), so perhaps it's time to include telephone care as part of this framework? Many long-term conditions are now reviewed via the telephone rather than in a face-to-face situation, so if this then forms part of QOF measurements, shouldn't we make sure that it is being done effectively and safely?

OOH services, however, at the time of writing, must adhere to the National Quality Requirement (NQR) standards. One of the NQR standards states that each person involved in the patient pathway (including call handlers and non-clinical staff) must be audited on a regular basis and through a random sample of interactions, along with 1% of patient experiences.

This standard is carried out in a variety of ways and is open to different interpretations, as it does not stipulate whether voice recordings, documentation or both should be audited. A 'random sample' could mean anything from listening to 50% of all call recordings, and reviewing the accompanying call record of each individual carrying out telephone triage, to reviewing only one call record/documentation and never listening to a single call voice recording. 'Regularly' could mean anything from auditing every week, to once every 2 years and everything in between!

This lack of clarity is both a help and a hindrance. Some organisations strive to provide evidence of monitoring taking place at frequent intervals to ensure the safety of their clinicians and operational efficacy. This in turn provides strong evidence for commissioners on the quality of the service, as well as the cost-effectiveness. I am also aware of a few organisations that are struggling to achieve a satisfactory standard of audit, or that are carrying out audits based on documentation alone and don't listen to call recordings at all. I believe that this is a major risk – sometimes the call documentation doesn't accurately reflect the actual phone call. To use this as a measure of quality could be totally inappropriate and potentially unsafe.

The quality of the auditor must also be considered. If the person responsible for carrying out the quality assurance hasn't been trained in using the audit tools, or does not have a clear understanding of what would constitute a safe and appropriate triage, what is the point of the audit?

If you have decided, however, that audit is the right thing for your organisation, how can you audit your calls?

8.2 How can you audit your calls?

In 2007 the Royal College of General Practitioners (RCGP) developed the Out of Hours Audit Toolkit to assist organisations to carry out audits in a comprehensive and structured way. The toolkit was designed to be applicable to doctors, nurses, call handlers and receptionists in both face-to-face and telephone assessments. It recommended that 1% of care episodes should be audited each quarter. However, the tool didn't stipulate what form the audit should take, but rather stated that it could involve auditing of voice recordings and/or call records for telephone encounters, which meant that it was open to interpretation.

The tool was updated and relaunched in 2011 as the Urgent and Emergency Care Clinical Audit Toolkit[2] and was developed further with the help of other organisations, including the Royal College of Paediatrics and Child Health and the College of Emergency Medicine. The philosophy and intent of the tool was admirable, as it was intended to be applicable across many providers of urgent and emergency care – a universal tool. However, in my opinion, this is also one of its drawbacks. Although the tool has undergone further development, the criteria for assessing the quality of an interaction (remember both face-to-face and telephone in one tool) remain the same. Furthermore, it was also intended to be used in a number of different areas, such as NHS Direct, NHS Pathways, ambulance services, emergency departments and OOH services. I believe that one tool cannot meet all the needs of such different organisations and roles, but I am aware that many organisations and practitioners use the tool to very good effect and have found it exceedingly useful. The toolkit is freely available online and is certainly a good starting point if you are new to clinical auditing of telephone consultations.

When it comes to auditing calls, you have the option of using tools such as those suggested previously, or simply providing feedback in a suitable environment, such as peer review or clinical supervision.

Wherever and however the audit is carried out, I would highly recommend that it's based on the voice recording (if available) *as well as* the patient's notes, if possible. An audit centred purely on the documentation of a call does not, in my opinion, provide enough information to allow a precise understanding of the phone call. Both parts of the interaction are needed for a detailed assessment of the phone call.

Many OOH service providers now use the revised tool as the basis for their audit, but, if the auditors haven't been trained in the clinical audit of telephone interactions, it can lead to inconsistent and inappropriate results – in other words, poor inter-rater reliability.

It is also important to note the role of 'statistics' in auditing. Numerous organisations measure the performance of their practitioners on quantitative information alone. In other words, they look at only the number of calls taken, how long their calls take, what their outcomes are and how all these figures compare with their peers or agreed targets. This is certainly a part of the analysis when it comes to audit, but it must always be balanced with qualitative information. How were the calls handled? Does the quality of the calls match the quantitative information? It's too easy to decide whether or not someone's practice is adequate (and safe) based on numbers alone. What is really important is how the call was managed between the triager and the caller. Was the outcome or length of call reasonable given the context?

The key to a good audit is to ensure that the auditors have been sufficiently trained in carrying out auditing and have access to robust criteria on which to base their assessment. For example, a statement such as 'Takes an appropriate history' within the RCGP tool could be interpreted in so many ways by different auditors. Conversely, we don't want to restrict the auditor's ability to offer individual judgement too much if it could help to improve practice.

Some organisations also believe that it's important that the auditors are actively involved in telephone triage, i.e. take calls themselves. I understand why this would be good practice, as they can be seen to be 'walking the walk' as well as 'talking the talk', but taking calls isn't always necessary, in my opinion. Knowing what constitutes a good call (via a good audit tool, for example), plus a thorough understanding of the operational and logistical background in which the calls are taken, is what is key. Alongside a good tool, a competency framework may also be a good resource on which to base your analysis of performance.

A competency framework for telephone assessments – do we need one?

Competence can be defined as 'The state of having the knowledge, judgement, skills, energy, experience and motivation required to respond adequately to the demands of one's professional responsibilities'.[3] When it comes to telephone triage, I believe that many clinicians are undertaking this role without the appropriate knowledge and skills, and one of the fundamental issues with telephone care is a lack of understanding and guidance about what is 'best practice'. If it's not regarded as a specialist clinical skill by governing bodies, why should clinicians be concerned about whether or not they have the ability to do this work? Neither the GMC nor the NMC has developed a framework that clinicians can look to for direction when delivering, or measuring, safe and competent practice (at the time of writing).

Some organisations have developed their own competency frameworks against which audits can be measured. However, this is rare. The lack of a framework means that, as clinicians, we have no defined standard against which we can measure our own skills or efficiencies. Areas that may need to be assessed include using the telephone and IT (information technology) systems, communication skills, clinical assessment (clinical safety), critical thinking, information gathering, decision making, negotiating skills, management planning and referral procedures – to name just some of the elements that constitute a good call!

Over the last few years, the lack of a framework has increasingly worried me. Therefore, I have developed a competency framework that could be applied to almost any clinical area in which patients are assessed over the phone (see Figure 8.1). This framework covers all of the areas that may need to be assessed and could be viewed as best practice guidance. For more information on clinical audit and this framework, visit my website, www. telelearning.co.uk.

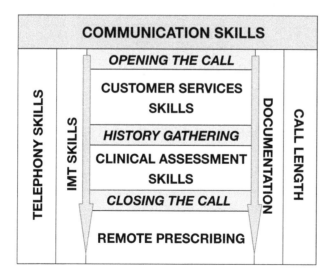

Figure 8.1 A competency model for telephone triage. IMT = information management and technology.

Following on from the development of the framework, I then progressed to writing audit tools based on the framework. The most comprehensive tool I have developed and implemented is based on a 'benchmark' approach. This details precisely what each criterion is observing and allows the auditor to mark from a score of 1 (no or little evidence) to 4 (best practice). Each score has an accompanying qualification for the auditor to mark against, and therefore measure against, reducing the chance of poor inter-rater reliability. The tool can also be viewed as best practice guidance for anyone new to telephone triage, or for those who are striving to be the very best at this complex, and diverse, type of work. For more information on this tool, see my website; Figure 8.2 shows a page from the tool.

On account of the time pressures in many organisations, however, a lengthy tool is not always well liked! Therefore, I have also developed a shorter tool, as a 'quick' safety tool that could be used in a basic way to quality assure calls. Figure 8.3 shows a page from that tool.

These tools are primarily based on having access to voice recordings or live monitoring, as well as documentation. They could be used with documentation alone, if necessary, by omitting the areas that relate to communication skills, for example, as these can only be quantified by hearing the call.

Standard 8	**Competency - Call Length and Time Managment** *(what is expected for appropriate time managment or length of the consultation given the nature of the call and resources available)*						
a	Demonstrates appropriate length of call and time management given nature of call						0
b	Call structure promotes safe and effective consultation times						0
	Total	**0**	**0**	**0**	**0**	**0**	**0**
	Score	**0%**	**0%**	**0%**	**0%**	**0%**	**0%**
	Overall Total For Call						

No Evidence - Call length is inappropriate given the nature of the call i.e too short and therefore presenting a risk to the patient or too long given the simplistic nature of the call and therefore preventing others accessing the service
Some Evidence - Call length is moderately shorter/longer than it could be given the nature of the call,but does not appear to present a risk to the patient or others trying to access the service at the time
Good Evidence - Call length appears appropriate for the nature of the call etc and makes some attempt to address the time the call is taking but may not manage to do so effectively
Best Practice - Call length has been actively managed throughout, whilst maintaining full engagement with caller and gathering sufficient history and ensuring others are not prevented from accessing the service

Figure 8.2 Sample page from the benchmarking audit tool.

	Closing Phase - Management Plan	0	0	0	0	0	0
9	Negotiates plan of action with caller, taking into account clinical picture, context and callers concerns						0
10	Clearly confirms final plan of action with caller						0
11	Provides safety netting advice,symptoms to watch out for relevant to outcome and call back instructions						0
	SCORE	0.00%	0.00%	0.00%	0.00%	0.00%	**0.00%**

Figure 8.3 Sample page from the basic 'safety tool'.

So, what else do you need to be able to carry out an audit, apart from training and tools?

8.3 What's needed to carry out quality assurance?

When carrying out clinical audit there are significant logistical and fiscal considerations that have an impact on the level and value of any quality assurance process. These are the main considerations when setting up quality assurance systems:

- access to calls or voice recordings
- access to call documentation or records
- access to an audit tool
- processes for collection of audit information
- storage and dissemination of audit information
- resources for carrying out the audit and giving feedback.

As well as the above requirements, you will also need to ensure that you have the following in place:

- training for auditors
- time to carry out the audit cycle
- administrative support
- feedback mechanisms for audit results.

Financial considerations include:

- the cost of training auditors
- the cost of carrying out audits
- the costs of 'replacing' or retraining poor practitioners identified through auditing.

So, as you can see, there is far more to clinical audit than simply having the right tool!

If you commit to a true quality assurance process and audit cycle, you will not only improve the care being delivered but also assist with the development of individuals, who may then go on to be experts in telephone triage. One of the foremost difficulties with telephone health care is a lack of standardisation among triagers. Auditing can help to calibrate practice, but another strategy that can help to achieve consistent practice is the use of protocols. Should we encourage more use of protocols?

References

1. Coleman A. Where do I stand? Legal implications of telephone triage. *Journal of Clinical Nursing* 1997; **6(3)**: 227–31.
2. Royal College of General Practitioners. *Urgent and Emergency Care Clinical Audit Toolkit*. London: RCGP, www.rcgp.org.uk/clinical-and-research/clinical-resources/urgent-and-emergency-care. aspx [accessed 28 September 2016].
3. Roach M.S. *The Human Act of Caring: a blueprint for the health professions*. Ottawa: Canadian Hospital Association Press, 1992.

Chapter 9

Protocols

9.1 Should you consider using protocols in telephone triage?

Using condition-specific protocols is definitely something worth considering to manage the risks in this clinical area. Training on telephone triage can certainly be enhanced by the use of these protocols. Another reason to consider the use of triage protocols is to achieve a level of consistency among a team, as protocols may help to standardise outcomes.

As suggested previously, the use of protocols could protect nurses from legal liability, and many nurses definitely prefer to triage with the support of a protocol – some even insist on it. However, most doctors don't use a protocol to assess patients, preferring to rely on their own clinical judgement, knowledge and experience.

Protocols can be bought 'off the shelf' or developed 'in house', and they are usually based on pattern recognition to provide better support for decision making. In addition, a good protocol should mimic the way the brain naturally solves problems.[1] Patients can be complex and symptoms are often ill defined, so you need a protocol that is sensitive enough to pick up the atypical and yet flexible enough to take into account the fact that sometimes patients and symptoms don't all fit neatly into a box. Finally, a protocol shouldn't force you to slavishly adhere to it – some level of discretion should be encouraged.

Nurses try to build a picture in their mind of the patient to compensate for the lack of visual clues, in a similar way to pattern recognition decision making. It has also been suggested that most clinical decisions made by experienced clinicians are based on a process akin to pattern recognition, rather than as a result of errors, such as the confirmation bias discussed as a risk.[2]

When I first began working in a telephone triage service, I had to use a clinical decision support system (CDSS). These computerised systems could be considered the most structured, and potentially confining, protocol that you can encounter. At first, however, having a CDSS was a huge relief and it was certainly a necessary support when I was new to triage. Many of the algorithmic protocols provided information on conditions that were unknown to me at the time, and they were not only helpful in guiding me to the outcome but they also improved my knowledge base immensely.

However, after working with several different CDSSs over the years, I noticed how many of my colleagues began to depend on them, to the point of overreliance, which can become a danger. They stopped critically thinking for themselves and became what was essentially a 'computer operator', or even an appointment clerk, rather than a high level clinician. If a protocol isn't available for the symptoms described, it can cause clinicians to 'panic' and mistriage, unless they also have the skills to triage without a specific protocol.

Protocols or a CDSS should neither take the place of formal instruction nor should they be treated as anything other than a decision support tool – and certainly not as a decision making tool. If clinicians depend too much on just what the protocol is 'asking', there is a risk that they can then ignore the tone of voice of the caller (a vital part of an assessment) or miss clues through lack of probing. They can be driven by the structure of the questions set, rather than really thinking about what they are being told. A protocol must be appropriate to the context in which it is being used to enhance clinicians' practice, without becoming a stumbling block. The goal is to create a protocol that is neither overly simplistic, in which case it will deal with calls too superficially, nor too complex, in which case it becomes cumbersome to use.

So, which is best? A protocol that you might develop in house, or one taken from an off-the-shelf book or a CDSS based on a computerised system?

9.2 Clinical decision support systems or protocols – what's right for you?

Before we consider what's right for you between a CDSS or bought or written protocols, it's important to note that, whatever type of system you choose, users must always rely on their clinical judgement to decide whether the response is positive or negative, especially when the protocol or system being used is based on branch logic. The biggest problem with a branch logic system is that patients and callers are not always simplistic in their answers (i.e. they don't only answer yes or no), and they will often respond with a vague answer that the clinician must then interpret, using the careful questioning techniques we have discussed. Overreliance on the system can be an issue – so, if the answer isn't clear cut, what does the triager do then? When patients, or their symptoms, don't fit neatly into a category, or provide a definitive answer, the real skill in telephone triage is to be able to work safely within those confines.

However, if you are expected to use some form of assessment tool, what are the strengths and weaknesses of the highly sophisticated computerised systems and protocols (either developed in house, or devised by others, and usually paper based, but not always) now available?

Clinical decision support systems

CDSSs are often criticised for being 'too restrictive' or turning triagers into 'computer operators', as I mentioned previously, but their greatest strength is that they enable you to keep the call structured. You must work your way through a series of questions in a restricted fashion, but in many cases this can also potentially minimise the risk of missing information. However, I have also witnessed users ignore vital information during calls, as they hadn't reached a certain question when the information was presented – an extreme case of the 'slavish' adherence we discussed in the previous section.

Some CDSSs are algorithmic in nature, such as the one used by NHS 111 and NHS Pathways (and previously NHS Direct), while others present various sets of questions, some of which may be mandatory, but most of which you can choose to ask or not and in whatever order you like. The positive responses in either case will then lead you to a suggested outcome. One of the skills required with these systems is picking the right protocol/algorithm title or set of questions and then recognising when the protocol/algorithm title isn't the right one and moving to the correct one promptly.

CDSSs commonly provide additional information for the user on the condition being assessed, allowing you to learn more about conditions or symptom patterns during the interaction and thereby developing your knowledge and expertise in what may have been an unfamiliar area.

As computer-based CDSSs are more restrictive and structured in their approach, there is a greater possibility of achieving standardised outcomes among users. Where individuals are using only their own clinical knowledge and experience to triage, or using a less restrictive protocol, it is likely to result in varied outcomes, as the questions asked can differ.

One of the biggest criticisms of systems such as NHS Direct and NHS 111 is that they often result in too high a level of outcome or are particularly risk averse. This perception, in my opinion, is often unfair. What is considered by many as a poor system, because of inappropriate outcomes, is often not the fault of the system but that of the individual clinician or user. In many cases that I have witnessed, the information had been presented by callers to clinicians but at a time when they weren't expecting it or hadn't asked about it. Clinicians would then ignore it, as they were too focused on the question at the time, rather than working outside the system. In addition, they wouldn't realise the importance of the information because they hadn't reached a certain point in the algorithm and would then miss a crucial issue.

Another concern that I had about CDSSs was that many users began to think that they knew better than the system, as it didn't always fill their needs, or they disliked having to work through questions that didn't seem relevant to them. They then bypassed the system, when it could actually have helped them.

The tendency to rely too much on the CDSS also became a major problem after a while. I felt that this was due, in part, to the operational demands on the clinicians. Having to take calls as quickly as they could, meant that some staff would simply go through an algorithm or set of questions as swiftly as possible. As these calls would then be referred to others for a face-to-face appointment outside their own service, there was little accountability, which may have contributed to the ease with which clinicians could slip into a 'soft triage'. I felt that the mundaneness of taking call after call, for long hours, was also a contributing factor that led to the lack of concern about their outcomes. When there was an adverse outcome, however, clinicians would often blame the system for failing to pick up on something, whereas, in my experience, the system was rarely the problem.

Protocols

Protocols that are bought off the shelf tend to be less restrictive and less informative than a CDSS, but they are a good deal cheaper! You could buy a pre-formatted protocol and then adapt it internally for your own use, i.e. add local information or pathways. Internally developed protocols are often 'guidance' rather than a protocol.

In the UK, there are very few books available that provide telephone triage condition-specific protocols. In the USA, there are a few more high-quality books that would certainly be beneficial to anyone new to triage, which are generally designed for nurses. If you are using one of these triage protocol books, please bear in mind that they are based on an accepted US clinical evidence base, which may not be regarded as best practice in the UK, and they won't mention NICE guidelines, for example. The terminology may not be the same either.

So what's best?

Having used a number of different CDSSs and externally and internally written protocols, which would I recommend? Or would I recommend any protocol at all? For me, using a CDSS and protocols most definitely helped when I was first triaging over the phone. I learnt so much about unusual conditions – knowledge that has stayed with me for decades. However, when I was allowed to 'free style', as I called it, i.e. triage using my own knowledge and experience (this is usually what most doctors would do), I also learnt what it was like to rely on my own clinical judgement – rather than on a protocol – using just my own questioning skills and understanding. I now prefer to do that, *but* I think that my confidence certainly increased and my knowledge base improved from learning about the structure of a call from a CDSS or protocol. For me, it isn't so much about being told what questions to ask but more about when to ask them in the flow of the call, how to prioritise questions and how to seek answers without asking closed and leading questions – one of the greatest problems with algorithmic systems.

Many services and practices now employ non-clinical staff to 'front end' calls that will then be passed on to a clinician for triage. These non-clinical staff are generally receptionists or call handlers, who are asked to 'filter out' calls that do not need clinical assessment and refer on those that do to clinical triage when necessary. Receptionists typically won't use any form of protocol, other than locally developed criteria. However, there are CDSSs that are designed for non-clinical staff. The largest user of a CDSS designed for non-clinical staff in the UK is NHS 111, which uses NHS Pathways; call handlers 'assess' using an algorithmic system specifically designed for these staff (there are different modules for each staff group). So, how important is this role of the receptionist in a telephone triage system?

References

1. Wheeler S. *Telephone Triage Protocols for Adult Populations.* (3rd edn). New York, NY: McGraw-Hill Medical, 2009.
2. Bradley C. Can we avoid bias? *BMJ* 2005; **330(7494)**: 784.

Chapter 10

The total triage system

10.1 How important is the role of the receptionist or call handler in telephone triage?

In many services, calls are initially handled by a non-clinician, typically a receptionist or call handler, before they appear on the call-back list for the clinician. There are exceptions to this in which the call is taken immediately by a nurse or doctor, but this isn't common in general practice.

How does the role of the receptionist affect the role of the triager, then? I believe that the initial handling of the call can have a dramatic impact on the triager for various reasons, which we will examine further in this chapter. I have developed my own training programmes for these staff, as the roles of the receptionist and the clinical triager are interlinked. It would be hazardous to underestimate the role of the person who first takes the call.

We know from research that 50% of patients in primary care can be managed safely over the phone, so why have we become so desperately short of appointments? We also know that some of the unmet demand is due to GPs' increased workload, declining numbers of GPs and increasing demands on GPs' time, all of which result in fewer available appointments. However, I also believe that some of the demand is due to patients who are taking appointments when they don't need them and, in many cases, when they don't need to go anywhere near a clinician, as their 'problem' can be addressed by other means. Patients are now booking appointments in advance 'just in case' they need them, because they are in such short supply – I know of two surgeries in which a weekly appointment was booked in case someone in the family needed it!

A few internal studies that I have seen in practices have shown that 20–33% of calls that come into the practice could be managed by receptionists or other administrative staff. In other cases, a patient may have asked for an appointment with a GP when a nurse, pharmacist or physiotherapist may have been able to help. Patients may also make an appointment with a GP when they should have used another healthcare resource such as A&E (the accident and emergency department) or a minor injury unit.

Given the pressure that today's primary care services are under, surgeries have begun to recognise that the receptionist is increasingly involved in managing the workload of the clinical team and some have developed the role even further – to the level of out-of-hours (OOH) call handlers or 'care navigators'. These staff are expected to carry out a form of 'triage' to identify the callers' needs and filter out those calls that don't need to go anywhere near a clinician. I prefer to think of this as 'signposting and prioritising' rather than 'triage', as they won't usually offer any clinical advice. They will, however, direct callers to the most appropriate place (signposting) or, if a patient requires urgent help, they will alert a clinician, as well as manage an obvious emergency over the phone by arranging an ambulance (prioritising).

To be able to signpost or prioritise correctly, the receptionist must find out the reason for the call or appointment. Most surgeries, however, will expect the receptionist to ask only the reason for the appointment or call-back if it's going on to a call-back queue, or it's a 'same day' or urgent appointment request, or there are only 'emergency' appointments left. In other words, the receptionist will ask the reason for the request only when appointments are in short supply or telephone triage seems appropriate but not when a routine appointment is available. This may seem reasonable, but, in my experience, many routine appointments are taken by patients who didn't require one.

I would even suggest that asking every patient about the reason for the appointment or contact is a necessary part of the receptionist's role, even if the patient wants a routine appointment in 4 weeks' time and there are several available. In my opinion, it's much safer and more efficient to have the receptionist ask the reason for the call and/or the reason the patient requires an appointment or call-back, to ensure that any appointments given are necessary and to direct patients to the right place. Let's not forget, too, that some patients will wait for the next available appointment when they should have been seen much sooner, therefore this system can prevent patients waiting too long and putting themselves at risk. If the receptionist is expected to signpost, he or she can only do that correctly by asking for the reason for the contact.

One last thing to note on asking the reason for the contact – *it's not what you ask, it's how you ask it!* We have already discussed the importance of tone of voice on the phone for the clinician, and the same applies to the reception-ist. Getting information from patients or callers when you aren't a clinician is difficult, and most receptionists haven't had any training on telephone com-munication and engagement, so you may want to consider sourcing some training for them, such as the training my company offers.

A call logged by the receptionist may contain quite a lot of detail about the reason for the call, which is then used by the clinician to prioritise when the call-back should be made. This makes a great deal of sense, especially when you have high call-back volumes and you know your patients and their demands well. Unfortunately, however, many surgeries still don't empower receptionists to ask for any information at all and simply want them to enter demographic information so that the triager can then call everyone back. So which system is best? I would suggest using your receptionists in the way that you feel is safest. If you have concerns about their skill set or their ability to ask the reason for the call, to signpost correctly and to engage with callers, you may want to limit their opportunities to elicit information, or to get some training in place to improve their competency. If your staff are used to asking the reason for the appointment or call-back, but in a limited capacity, you might want to consider extending this to all calls, but ensure that they are supported by training if necessary.

The role of the receptionists is crucial to the success of some service delivery models, such as the total triage model, but what is this model really about?

10.2 What is total triage and should you use it?

'Total triage' is one of the service delivery models that practices are now look-ing to in order to manage patient demand and maximise capacity. It operates in the same way as OOH services in that, when patients phone the surgery and request an appointment, they are told that a clinician will call them back first. If a face-to-face appointment is still required *after the triage*, the clinician will arrange that *with* the patient, usually that day. No matter when patients want to be 'seen', they are asked to contact the surgery on the day and they will talk to a clinician first before an appointment is allocated. If the system is effective and the triage is also effective, typically only 30–40% of patients are seen after triage. At the same time, access (or contacts) can be improved by up to 50%.

The receptionists allocate mainly telephone appointments and add to the call-back list, instead of booking in face-to-face appointments. There are some exceptions: typically, around 10% of patients will automatically require a face-to-face appointment, such as new baby checks, contraceptive pill checks or mental health reviews for vulnerable patients who may not be able to make contact themselves, but generally 90% of patients can be triaged over the phone first.

So does this model really work and should you consider using it? I have personally worked with surgeries that have implemented this system, and it has been so successful that it has had a staggering effect on the staff and the patients. Although they are dealing with more patients on a daily basis, they aren't working harder – just smarter, as the saying goes! The clinicians manage their own workloads and each day is fluid, as the appointment book is almost empty at the start of the day. It can be extremely liberating, as clinicians can see patients whenever it's convenient, or do home visits at any time, rather than just at lunch time, as is the norm. The receptionists no longer have to argue or negotiate with patients about what is urgent or not, or if they should be squeezed in as an extra appointment. The patients quickly learn that they will be given an appointment on the day that they contact the surgery, no matter what time they ring in, and therefore they don't have the stress of trying to get through as soon as the surgery opens in the morning or the fear of being too late to get a same-day appointment. Everyone goes home at the end of the busiest days with a sense of satisfaction and a smile – honestly, it can be that successful.

The total triage system can and does work, no matter what your patient demographic. However, I have also seen it fail spectacularly, usually for one of three reasons:

1   poor preparation and planning – among staff and patients
2   receptionists not filtering properly and just using the triage call-back list as a bit of a dumping ground, creating more work for the clinicians than is necessary
3   clinicians not triaging effectively and converting too many calls to a face-to-face consultation after the triage thereby increasing their workload.

One other thing that the system depends on is a cohesive team. If anyone isn't keen on triaging, or if any of the receptionists prefer the old system in which they were 'in charge' of allocating appointments, it's easy for the system to be sabotaged.

If these things can be avoided or managed, I would definitely recommend this way of working, but, if you are considering moving to this model, please plan carefully. Premature implementation will result in too many problems and you will think that the system doesn't work when in fact it could. So what do you need to consider when moving to this service delivery model?

10.3 What's needed to implement a total triage system?

When it comes to preparation, there's a huge amount that you have to plan and think through before implementation. Rushing into implementation will almost certainly result in failure, as discussed previously. You need to know that everyone is on board with this new way of working, as it will mean a big change for all involved and, as we know, not everyone is comfortable with change. Do your research into how others have managed and take your time to think and plan to save you as much stress as possible after launch day.

Planning for a total triage model

Below are just some of the things that you will need to consider.

- How will you communicate with patients about the system?
- How will you use your telephone message (if you use one)?
- Do the receptionists require training on the new system and how they communicate on the phone?
- Do the clinical staff require training on telephone triage?
- What do you call the call-backs – telephone triages, telephone consultations or telephone appointments or something else?
- Should you use headsets or handsets?
- Have you got an adequate number of phone lines?
- How will you allocate the phone calls as they come in?
- How will you allocate the face-to-face appointments following the call-back?
- Have you planned your workforce capacity?
- How will you set up your appointment times for the face-to-face appointments that are exempt from the triage system?
- How will you manage and identify pre-booked appointments and follow-up appointments?
- How will you manage your internet appointment system?
- How will you manage 'walk-ins'?
- What will you do for patients who are hard of hearing, don't have a phone or are unable to use a phone?
- How will you manage requests for home visits?
- How will you plan for 'launch day'?

This is not an exhaustive list! As you may have guessed by now, the system takes a great deal of prior planning, championing and preparation at all levels. You will need to be primed to make changes and tweaks, on almost a daily basis, until you think it is working well and in a way that everyone is comfortable with. Having said that, be careful of tweaking too much – you must give it time to settle in – and avoid being too reactive.

If you do decide to consider this model, I would urge you to consult other practices that have been successful and learn from their mistakes, or perhaps use a consultant who offers more than just data-gathering information. Although this is extremely useful, the data are only one small part of the success of the system. Be wary of companies that advocate 3-minute triage times for all calls as a basis for working out your capacity planning. Although this is entirely possible with some of your patients, and when a full assessment isn't required, e.g. test results, medication queries, etc., when it comes to doing a good assessment, offering self-care and patient education, I would encourage you to take an average of 5 minutes as your starting point. If you have read all my advice on how to take a call, I hope that you realise that many of your calls will take more than 3 minutes, especially if you reach an outcome of self-care and you want to achieve all the benefits of telephone work. If you aren't prepared to take the time, or you convert too easily to a face-to-face outcome, there is no point in telephone triage. The time savings and improved access can be achieved only through safe and effective triage.

So, as you can see over the course of this book, there is far more to telephone triages and consultations (just in case you still prefer to think of them as separate entities) than most clinicians suspect. From the purpose of the phone call, to an outcome that is right for the patient, for the clinician and for the resources that are available, there is so much to consider that it can seem like too much. Surely, it's easier just to carry on with the system that we and our patients have been used to over the decades – patients make an appointment to see the GP or nurse and, fingers crossed, one will be available when they want it? In today's mobile society and consumer-driven culture, I don't think that the 'old system' is sustainable, or indeed acceptable. Why should patients have to come into the surgery when they may lose time off work, and therefore salary, or have to bring five children in at the same time, when it is something that could be managed over the phone? Why should clinicians have to work more than 12 hours a day, just to get through all the 'extras' that have been added because there aren't enough appointments? If telephone assessments can help to ease the burden on the NHS and the clinicians, as well as make life easier for the patients and provide more timely intervention, surely we owe it to ourselves and our patients to make sure that we are carrying out this work safely and effectively? I earnestly hope that our governing bodies, the NHS, training institutions and even the government realise the benefits that using the phone to provide care can bring – but only when it's done well.

References

1. Bunn F, Byrne G, Kendall S. The effects of telephone consultation and triage on healthcare use and patient satisfaction: a systematic review. *British Journal of General Practice* 2005; **55(521)**: 956–61.

Chapter 11

Summary

It isn't easy to summarise all the learning that this book is intended to provide, but I hope that the following will help to highlight the key points in each chapter.

Triage versus consultations

We clarified that, for the purposes of this book, calls that don't involve a form of assessment, or those not based in a clinical episode, such as sick note requests, repeat prescription requests, test results, information sharing, etc. (routine work), should not be considered a triage or a consultation. We are referring only to those calls that require a clinical assessment of new or ongoing symptoms.

These calls can be referred to as a triage in some cases and a consultation in others. Many clinicians consider a telephone triage to be different from a telephone consultation but, in practical terms, the work done by the clinician is exactly the same – you ask some questions, rule out/in acute signs and symptoms by levels of priority and reach an outcome according to the priority, or not, as the case may be.

However, I believe that our approach to the call can vary according to whether we are expecting a 'triage' (a quick, precise signposting) or a 'consultation' (an in-depth discussion, potentially resulting in self-management and requiring more time). Removing the need to classify calls as either a triage or a consultation, and viewing the interaction simply as a telephone assessment, may prevent you second guessing what the call will be about, what the outcome might be and how long it will take. Your actions in either a triage or a consultation are likely to be the same, but predetermined actions are a real risk when it comes to the calls. Another of the biggest dangers when taking calls is that of time pressure. This can have a dramatic impact on the call, so we need to be mindful of the time taken, without it dictating our actions. Time pressures lead to rushing the call, which in turn affects the information we might collect, as well as our tone of voice.

Chapter 1 also looked at the benefits and risks of telephone work. There are enormous benefits to be had, but only when the triage is done well. Recognising where the risks lie will help you to manage those risks and decide if a telephone interaction is the safest option.

The purpose of telephone triage

Understanding the purpose of the call and what you are trying to achieve is crucial. It will help you enormously with your decision making. The aims of a call are summarised in the following three principles.

---

1 *determine if the patient needs to be seen*
2 *if the patient does need to be seen, define when, by whom and where*
3 *ensure that the caller is satisfied with the interaction.*

One of the reasons that many calls are overly long or complex is because the clinician is focused on diagnosing. This is not to say that this isn't important, as you need a differential diagnosis in order to decide whether or not someone needs a face-to-face consultation. The primary aim, however, is to determine the need for further assessment, not to ensure the correct diagnosis. Once you know that a patient needs to be seen, your call should reach its conclusion, unless any further questions are required to determine the place of contact, or the level of care. To acquire the best quality information and an accurate history, along with caller compliance at the end of the call, the triager must engage the caller throughout, and how to do this was discussed in detail in Chapters 2 and 3.

The importance of understanding how the patient perceives telephone consultations must be acknowledged. Why would patients or carers trust us to help care for them or their relatives, or give advice, when we haven't been able to see them, touch them or listen to anything other than their voices? Building confidence in the caller relies on our ability to communicate and listen effectively, especially in the absence of visual confirmation or responses such as body language.

The three key stages to call taking

The majority of clinical assessment calls will involve three stages: the introduction, the information-gathering stage and the management plan. It's important to work your way through these stages in the correct order. It will ensure that you address issues such as confidentiality and that you take a history in a structured way to reach the most suitable outcome within the shortest time possible. It reduces the risk of poor information gathering, or alienating the caller, which in turn makes compliance less likely at the end of the call. In Chapter 4 we discussed how you work your way through each of these stages to complete the call with an appropriate level of safety netting – probably the most important feature of any call, but particularly when you are advising self-management.

History taking and decision making vary among professionals. We know that doctors and nurses, as well as experts and novices, make decisions in different ways, but understanding the three principles and adhering to them whenever possible should help you to reach your decisions in the shortest time frame.

Managing closure

Many clinicians struggle to decide when a call should finish or worry about whether they have done enough: 'Should I have asked more about…?' or 'Perhaps I should offer to call them back to see how they are doing?'. Understanding your role as a telephone triager and how to prepare for the unexpected whenever you can will provide you with tools and techniques for managing difficult calls. Clear communication with the patient, the receptionist and the clinician is needed to ensure that the next steps have been agreed and understood. Keeping the receptionist in the loop will make future contacts streamlined for both the patient and the clinician.

If callers or patients refuse to take your advice, the main point to consider is whether they are making an informed decision. Have you clearly explained why you have reached your decision? Have you described and discussed alternative solutions if the caller is unable to comply? At times, you will need to override the caller's decision, e.g. if there is a safeguarding issue or if you suspect diminished capacity. If the patient is an adult and fully capable of accepting or declining our advice, as long as we have been clear in our understanding and communicated our reasoning, callers can always choose not to accept our advice. In Chapter 5 we looked at the issues you may face when callers refuse to take your advice, but it is always worth talking to your indemnity provider for further information on where your responsibility lies when there is a conflict between you and your caller.

Documentation and record keeping

We must be careful about how much we document, as this in itself can be the cause of overly long interactions. The documentation principles that apply to face-to-face consultations are the same for telephone consultations. However, we need to replace any clinical findings that we would normally have had the opportunity to discover in a physical examination with a 'verbal' examination. In Chapter 7 I suggested documentation criteria to help minimise your documentation, while maximising the applicability of the content. The ultimate aim in record keeping is to have call voice recordings available, but this isn't always possible in many areas of work. Where recordings can be made, we know that complaints and incidents are far more easily dealt with. Training and development is reinforced through the use of voice recordings and they can moderate both the caller's and the clinician's behaviour. As voice recordings are relatively non-invasive, I would highly recommend them. Be careful, however, to observe the correct legal requirements when recording calls. Listening to your own calls is the best form of personal development.

Medicolegally, voice recordings are admissible in court, but, even when voice recordings are possible, the primary record remains your electronic record. The safest way to view your record keeping is to remember the mantra, 'If it's not written down, it didn't happen.'

Quality assurance

The quality assurance of telephone interactions is still in its infancy in general practice, but it's becoming much more commonplace through the use of call recording equipment and certainly in out-of-hours services, where there are National Quality Requirement standards in place. In Chapter 8 we looked at why you might wish to consider carrying out some sort of quality assurance of your calls and what you would need to consider logistically. If you are intending to audit your calls, or are the subject of clinical audit, it's advisable to question the tools and skill set of those carrying out the audit. Is it based on a competency framework? Can you develop best practice guidelines to support safe and effective telephone triage?

Protocols

Depending on your background and clinical role, you may or may not be required to use triage protocols that are condition specific, such as 'Back pain in an adult' or 'Fever in a child under 10'. In Chapter 9 we discussed when protocols can be useful and when they can hinder your assessment. There are various types of protocols – from those bought 'off the peg' to more structured systems, such as a clinical decision support system, like those used by NHS 111. Knowing where the limitations lie in using any of these protocols is key, and learning not to rely on them too much, or ignore them, is equally important. Patients unfortunately don't fit into simple 'yes or no' response categories. One of the biggest risks of some protocols is that they can't pick up on every possible thing that a caller may disclose or the non-verbal clues that a triager may need to decipher. The best protocols are designed to support the triager, while allowing their own critical thinking, knowledge and experience to come into play.

The role of the receptionist and the total triage model

Most calls that reach the clinician have been initially dealt with by a non-clinical member of staff such as a receptionist, care navigator or call handler, although it is still possible in some services that the call could go directly to the clinician. However, if a receptionist or other non-clinician has handled the call first, that can have a direct impact on the role of the triager. Workload can be reduced or increased by the initial handling of the call, so it's necessary to keep looking at how we support these staff. Do you have protocols in place to assist their handling of calls? If you are running a total triage system, the role of the receptionists is critical to its success. In Chapter 10 we studied what you need to consider when initiating and operating this type of access system, as well as the risks and benefits. For many practices and clinical commissioning groups, this type of access model is becoming increasingly popular but, once again, it relies on the skills of the initial call-handling staff to filter out inappropriate call-backs, as well as the skill of the triager, to ensure that the rate of conversion to face-to-face consultations is appropriate. Just doing telephone triage is not the key – getting it right is!

Final words

Throughout this book I have attempted to demystify the complex and often daunting world of telephone triage and consultations. Telephone interactions carry inherent risks, and it requires the continuous calculation of those risks to decide when calls should conclude and when they should continue.

Telephone triage and consultations can be far less overwhelming to those who are nervous of assessing and advising when they aren't able to see the patient if you develop your own call structure and break the call down into stages. Underpinning this process, however, there has to be an understanding of the communication skills needed when you can't see your patient or caller. This will help you to manage the call, and keep the caller sufficiently engaged, so that you reach a mutually agreeable and appropriate outcome.

By having a clear process and structure for your calls, while remembering that the primary purpose is to determine the need for face-to-face consultations, and not to diagnose, you will be able to achieve more efficient and rewarding calls.

My very last point of advice would be to always make sure you are really listening to your caller – as the title of this book suggests! By truly listening, you will become a better triager.

Index